Published by Gratitude Healing Arts, LLC
ISBN: 978-0-578-24586-7

Cover Art: Nicole Rachelle Keane, 2020
Illustrations and Calligraphy: Nicole Rachelle Keane, 2021, 2020, 2019
Photography: Open Source; but for the photo of the Trees at the end of the *zhi* chapter, ©Carletto Del Monaco

This manual is not intended to be used in diagnosis or treatment of any health condition, in any way, unless the user is licensed by the regulatory jurisdiction where they practice to provide such services of diagnosis and treatment. The author and publisher do not endorse self diagnosis or treatment by non-medical professionals.

For more information visit www.gratitudehealingarts.com.

"WHEN WE ARE IN A STATE OF *GRATITUDE*, WE ARE BATHED IN CUES OF *SAFETY*."

- DR. STEPHEN PORGES

5% from the sale of each and every electronic copy of this manual, purchased directly from the website www.gratitudehealingarts.com, will be distributed to a non profit that assists people recovering from trauma or addiction, or directly to an individual that has been affected by physical or emotional trauma. This donation is intended to be put toward lifting and supporting the human nature, through gratitude and ease, on the path of healing and resilience.

If you have purchased this manual on another platform and would like to make a donation that will go toward this mission, please visit www.gratitudehealingarts.com.

THIS MANUAL IS DEDICATED TO *LING*

靈氣

AND THE HEALING OF DISTORTED MASCULINE ENERGY THROUGH THE RISE AND SUPPORT OF THE DIVINE FEMININE

...AND NAMAH

“Whether or not you can observe a thing depends upon the theory you use.

It is the theory which decides what can be observed.”

– Albert Einstein

Contents

The Wheel turns and shapes;

Formed by Awareness of Touch;

Ideas Reformed.

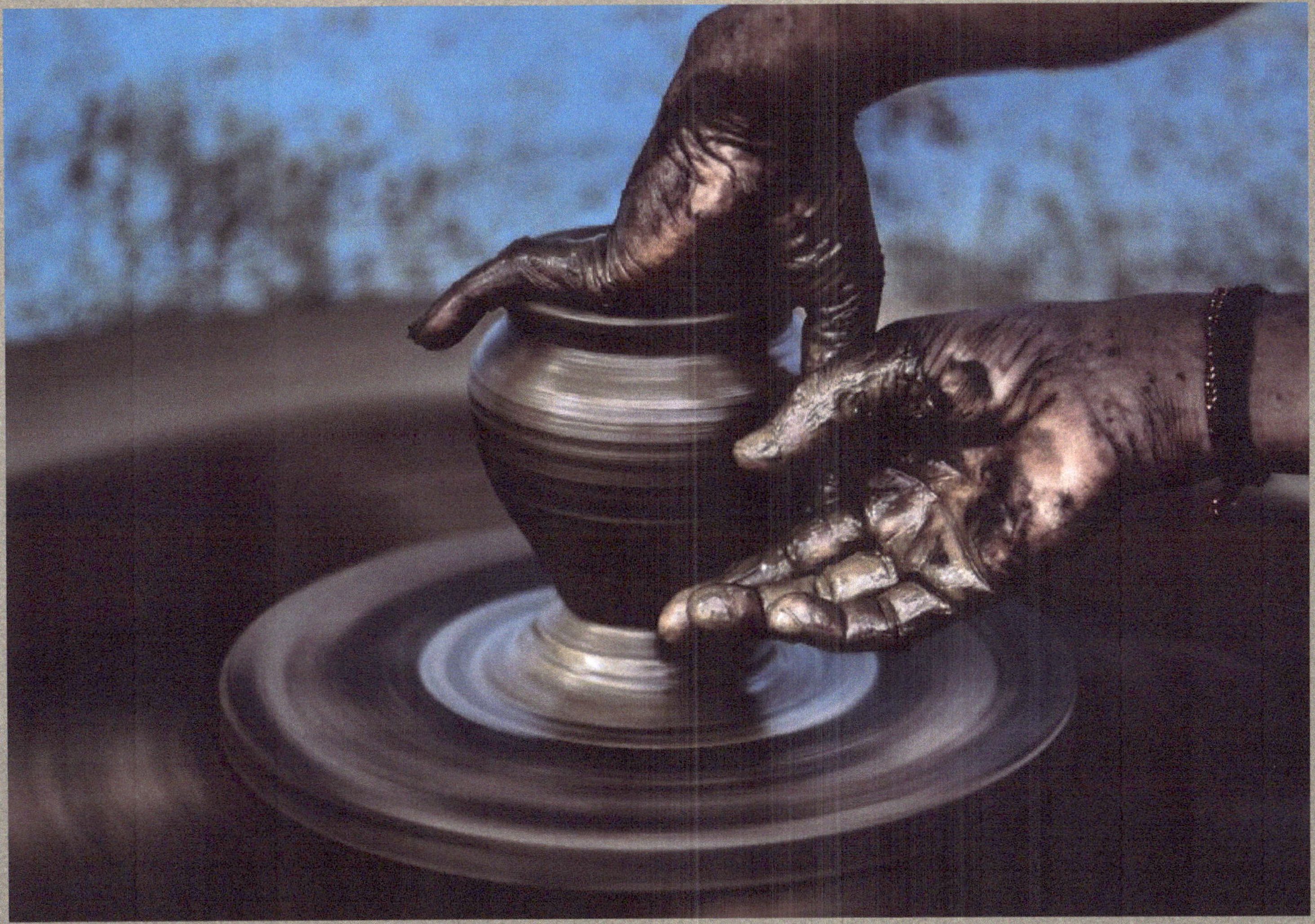

Author's Note

I hope to offer enough introductory information within this publication to make it interesting to all who venture into its pages. With one hand, this publication touches on the paradigm shifting *Polyvagal Theory*, a modern construct based on new perspectives of the human Autonomic Nervous System (ANS). The other hand reaches toward ancient ways of healing, toward patterns and perspectives offered by a view of the body as an ecosystem, in relation to the holographic nature of the Universe. If the learning curve seems steep for you as an Observer, please be patient with yourself and venture slowly. Taking time to digest the information I have brought into these pages is essential. These pages touch into a world that many trained professionals have spent years of study within. Simply being open to exploring this world is the only requirement. The illustrations contained within these pages are meant to serve as inspirations for healing meditation and reflection. I hope you enjoy this journey.

To the trained professionals that are familiar with the disciplines of study described in these pages, this manual is intended to be a practical tool for the integration of the *Polyvagal Theory,* with the evolving perspectives of *Five Element* Asian medical theory. It will also serve as an introduction to a technical manual therapy curriculum called Elemental Manual Meridian Theory and Techniques (EMMT). The purpose of EMMT is to bring together manual release of energetic and physical restrictions within the anatomy of the body, in order to affect the physiology of the body and ANS. The ideas presented here may be integrated and applied to other modern medical disciplines and esoteric philosophies, and are intended to be a bridge between ancient and modern theories of healing within the human design. Detailed discussions of the specific anatomy and physiology of the concepts presented in this manual, as well as techniques for clinical application, will be available within the classes of the EMMT curriculum.

- Nicole Rachelle Keane, MS LMT

"When one begins to carry out one's decision, care must be taken so that everything can proceed in a comfortable, relaxed manner. Too much must not be demanded of the heart. One must be careful that, quite automatically, heart and energy are co-ordinated. Only then can a state of quietness be attained. During this quiet state the right conditions and the right space must be provided…All entanglements must be put aside; one must be detached and independent… danger arises if too much trouble is taken. I do not mean that no trouble is to be taken, but the correct way lies in keeping equal distance between being and non-being. If one can attain purposelessness through purpose, then the thing has been grasped. Now one can let oneself go, detached and without confusion, in an independent way. "

The Secret of the Golden Flower - Translation by Richard Wilhelm

The Observer will notice that many of the quotes within this book, referencing Classical, as well as current texts regarding the *Five Elements*, are taken out of context… and when applied to the different perspective provided by the *Polyvagal Theory*, still ring very true. This is a synchronicity that begs further contemplation, and certainly application, within the new areas of wellness that humanity is evolving toward.

Within this manual I refer to the spirit affiliations differently than the interpretations of most Classical texts. The spirit affiliation for each element is noted with a lower case letter, while the Spirit (proper noun) is referred to with an upper case letter. The Spirits have a holographic resting place within the organ of the preceding element and spirit affiliation. For instance the spirit affiliation for the *Earth* element is *shen;* while the Spirit that nests within the Heart, of the *Fire* element, is *Shen*.

DEFINITIONS OF COMMON ASIAN MEDICAL TERMS

I would like to offer the person unfamiliar with common Asian medical terms an opportunity to read this text without having to look too many concepts up, as such I have referenced several terms in this forward.

The concepts of the Spirits: *Zhi*, *Hun*, *Shen*, *Yi*, and *Po*, will be described as paramount content, and their meaning, as it applies to the concepts presented in this manual, should be apparent through explanation within each chapter.

Yin - *Identifying as Feminine energy, receptive, soft, can become distorted from its Divine nature by trauma and stress. The opposite polarity to yang.*

Yang - *Identifying as Masculine energy, initiatory energy, active; can become distorted from its Divine nature by trauma and stress. The opposite polarity to yin.*

Tao - *The Way of awareness; all that is within that is constantly flowing out; all that is without that is constantly moving toward and passing within.*

Te - *Original nature, Virtue, Intuition; having Integrity through one's path in life.*

Wu - *The shamanic spirit of emptiness that contains the mysterious wisdom of the Universes. The vacuum of non-being.*

Yuán - *Origin; the original nature of something that spontaneously flows into being.*

Wúwéi - *A state of actively receiving; doing without doing; being without being. A place within from which radical acceptance of what is without arises.*

Wēijī - *A turning point on the path of transformation and healing. The moment of inspiration. A crux point. A point of reflection.*

Hùndùn - *Chaos. A state of disorder from where transformation occurs; raw form before balance. Primordial Chaos.*

Tan - *Alchemy. The negentropic transformation of energy within a system.*

Yu - *To heal. To meet something on the level it is at, in that moment, and supportively initiate healing.*

Shen - *Concept in classical Asian medical theory that relates to spirit, or the Five Spirits. Translated literally as 'expansion of the Divine,' it is the energy of Divine creativity and light extending through human experience. Shen as a proper noun refers to the Spirit that resides within the Heart; shen, as a spirit affiliation, rests supportively within the Earth element.*

Qì - *Energy, Intention, Intuition. The functions of qì are movement, protection, transformation, retention, and warming. Qì is intimately related to the Asian medical concept of Blood. The Force; "It's an energy field created by all living things. It surrounds us and penetrates us; it binds the galaxy together." Obi-Wan Kenobi*

Jing - *Primal essence that is instilled within our being as the embryo develops in utero. It arises as the primitive Biliary and Stomach projections differentiate in fetal development. The Liver and Stomach emanate jing toward the Kidneys. Jing is responsible for seating Qì within the Kidneys.*

Ling *- The aspect of spirit, or shen, that makes manifest the Divine into form, effecting change in the Earth realm. The process and power of receiving the energy of Divine purpose, and actioning it into being.*

Shēng Cycle *- A classical model of healing used in Five Element Asian medical theory that is based on seasons of entropy and negentropy. The yin and yang energies rotate and exchange in life-death-life cycles, focusing on creation, generation, nourishment, and consumption; with qì flowing clockwise through the elements.*

K'o Cycle *- A classical model of healing used in Five Element Asian medical theory that is based on control and limitation of life's energies. The energy of this cycle crosses the Five Element wheel from one point to another, creating a star pattern.*

Xiè Cycle *- A classical model of healing used in Five Element Asian medical theory that is based on reduction, draining, and exhaustion of life's energies. The energy of this cycle flows counter-clockwise within the Five Element wheel, in opposition to the Shēng Cycle. This cycle can be used to assess the affects of trauma and stress on the human ecosystem.*

*__Tan Cycle__ - *A philosophical treatment model used in various healing practices involving the Five Element theory of balance and harmony within the body. This cycle involves correlations made to universal characteristics of external ecosystems. The Tan Cycle, as a treatment model, is based on counter-clockwise flowing qì, holographic representations of the spirit affiliations to reference quantum energy potentials, and negentropic principles of lifting and supporting energies within the system. This treatment model focuses on achieving balanced Masculine (yang) and Feminine (yin) energies, as well as functional application of anatomy and physiology, to create transformative healing potentials within the Autonomic Nervous System.*

*__Yu Angles__ - *A philosophical treatment model that compliments the Tan Cycle. Each of the Five Elements refer to angular correlations with the two elements across the Tan Cycle, creating an angle, originating from each element. Healing potentials are based on the supportive characteristics and interactions of each element that help resolve physical and energetic disfunction within the Autonomic Nervous System. If there are physical or energetic symptoms of disfunction within an element, the Observer would look toward the two elements at Yu angle from the element of focus for potential options of healing, support, and assistance with resolving balance and restoring function. Using Yu angles for treatment is intended to support the counter-clockwise flow of qì within the Tan Cycle.*

**** denotes new terms created by the author for this publication***

"At this critical point in human history, moving through the *Wēijī* means finding a way to reintegrate the realms that dualism split apart - not by turning back to an outmoded wholeness, but by discovering a new, more complex integrity. It means developing a new way of honoring the spirits that animate the energies of life on our planet so that we can consciously recognize and relate to them, not as disembodied entities, but as aspects of the divine that exist here and now, in our own being and our daily lives."

-Lori Eve Dachar, 'Five Spirits'

THE EVOLUTION OF PRACTICAL APPLICATION OF THE FIVE ELEMENTS

The framework of the social structure of modern times is quite different than that of the Taoist sages of 4,000-5,000 years ago, as well as the Chinese philosophers of 2,000 years ago, that contributed to the genesis of the current *Five Element* system of Asian medical theory.

Moreover, humanity has existed within a mostly patriarchal societal context since the beginning of what we currently think of as the written language and historical methods recording. As such, many of the subtle essences of the original theories may have gotten lost or misconstrued in over the ages through translation... And no doubt, some bits of insight were never written down, or may have been 'lost' within oral tradition, or cultural secret.

These ways of viewing the *Five Elements,* as presented in the concepts I will bring forward, have a bit of a different flare. I am not attempting to confuse the Observer, nor discredit what has come before, nor attest to any inadequacy; "traditional" theory is just viewed from a different lens than through which I have seen, and can indeed coexist, as the practitioner sees relevant within their clinical practice.

These concepts presented in this book are simply ideas, a *Way* of doing things. It is the Observer's opportunity to decide what resonates for their practice.

"Diversity emerges as the natural expression of balanced relationship between human will and the will of heaven. The will of heaven is continuous, creative, evolutionary change. Humans formulate ways of knowing that consist of models and systems. Newtonian physics, quantum mechanics, and the five-element system are examples. These models represent the human attempt to understand the earth and the nature of our lives upon it. It is human nature to cling to these models and the momentary stability that they appear to afford amid continuous change. Our models remain static, and as we build them into towering monolithic structures whose foundations consist of assumptions and meanings we create, the true nature of life continues to evolve and outgrow them. The edge of the creative change is always just beyond the grasp of our deepest intuition. The momentary stability afforded by such models is an illusion because the essential nature of life remains chaotic and unknowable. Models are tools, elaborate stories, and we must recognize them as such. Diversity is what emerges when individuals are each able to embrace the freedom to create their own mythology while simultaneously allowing others that same freedom. For the sage, all stories are created equal inasmuch as they empower the creative flow of life."

– Lonny Jarret, 'Nourishing Destiny'

THE *POLYVAGAL THEORY*

This manual is intended to speak of a shift from the traditional view of the *Five Element* spirit affiliations, toward a reinterpretation of the traditional Eastern concepts of the Spirit; an interpretation that integrates the information that we have come to know about how trauma and stress affect the Autonomic Nervous System (ANS), and how our bodies regulate essential functions such as digestion, breathing, and heart rate.

The ideas for this shift, and the creation of a new framework to approach healing the energetic and physical body in clinical practice, have come to me from my observations within meditation; my personal clinical observations of how energy is stored and moves through the body; as well as my research into the nuances of the physiological and psychological implications of the paradigm shifting *Polyvagal Theory*, developed by Dr. Stephen Porges, and put into practice by various clinical disciplines.

The *Polyvagal Theory* opens the door to a new world of quantum physiology involving the *Five Elements*.

I recommend reading the work of Dr. Porges, as well as the work of Deb Dana, for familiarizing yourself with the broader concepts and implications of the work of Dr. Porges and his colleagues. For a general orientation that will be helpful to the Observer when reading the material presented hereafter, I will provide some brief explanation, and further definition throughout the text, as concepts are discussed in detail relative to each of the *Five Elements*.

The *Polyvagal Theory* has given the medical world a way of understanding physiological and emotional imbalance in a much more nuanced way. This perspective includes two divisions of Parasympathetic function, and the well known Sympathetic branch of the ANS; as well as a reasoning that the nervous system processes and responds to stimuli in a hierarchical manner, based on how the ANS evolved, as humans differentiated from other species, advancing into nuanced social behavior. As this evolution has progressed, so has our experience of stress.

The *Polyvagal Theory* has been used widely in the disciplines of Clinical Behavioral Psychology, Social Work, and Occupational Therapy. It is commonly applied when working with children and adults that have behavioral and developmental disabilities, or history of trauma.

Simply: Poly means "many" and Vagal, refers to the Vagus nerve.

Historically called the Pneumogastric Nerve; named from the Latin for "Wandering," this nerve is the key to a lot of chronic health issues, due to the great impact that it has on the Autonomic functions of the body, as well as its role in systemic inflammation.

The Autonomic Nervous System is a bi-directional system that is very influenced by visceral feedback and emotional processing. The Vagus nerve (CN X) is the main method of communication within this system. The *Polyvagal Theory* notes that there are many regulating structures that influence the Autonomic functions governed by the Vagus nerve. The entire complex of interconnected neural fibers of all the Cranial nerves, that weave to and from the Cranial nerve nuclei within the Medulla, have an impact on the regulation ability of the Vagus.

The *Polyvagal Theory* helps explain the psychological and physiological impacts of trauma, and has helped to create different types of therapy, across many disciplines, that honor the role of the Autonomic Nervous System as we move through States of protection, withdrawal, and connection, in an ongoing quest for safety.

The Vagus nerve is not merely one long, wandering nerve; it is made up of many different nerve fibers that send information

TO the Brain, ***FROM*** the visceral organs (***afferent fibers***), as well as…

FROM the Brain ***TO*** the visceral organs (***efferent fibers***)

You can think of it as a fiber optic cable, or bundle of various nerve fibers, some myelinated (insulated), some unmyelinated, on which information travels at very fast speeds, with connections to other Cranial nerves, a relay system of nuclei in the Brainstem, and a control center of higher order neurons and nuclei within the Brain.

Together, this system is the Polyvagal Complex…and it is very complex. The function of the Vagus involves 80% *afferent* communication, physical and energetic information, coming *from* the body *to* the Brain, and only 20% of information that travels on the nerve complex is *efferent*, going *from* the Brain *to* the body.

In this way, the health of our external environment, as well as the health of our internal visceral ecosystem, influences our emotions and actions. Information about state shifts within the body is sent through neural connections to Cranial nerve nuclei in the Brainstem, and then further to areas of the Cortex and the Limbic system for processing and integration.

The Ventral Vagus is the myelinated Vagus, and controls Autonomic function *above* the Diaphragm, also sending a small amount of fibers to aid in function *below* the diaphragm.

The Dorsal Vagus, is the *un*myelinated Vagus, and sends fibers to viscera *below* the diaphragm, with only a very small portion of *un*myelinated fibers joining the Ventral Vagus, to innervate the Autonomic Nervous System above the Diaphragm.

Psychologically, the Ventral Vagus is involved with self-regulating and co-regulating the nervous system through healthy emotional responses and fostering pro-social behavior.

The Dorsal Vagal complex is the more primitive nervous system, and is responsible for the immobilization response to stress and trauma, that can take on many different physical and emotional forms.

In order to truly understand how the body responds to trauma and stress, we must have a perspective of the entire landscape that we are working within… The Vagal complex reaches far and wide within the internal environment, and the *Five Elements* exist within the internal environment as well. We are immersed in the processes of our internal Nature, finding balance.

As a matter of sensory perception, the entire Polyvagal complex informs our nervous system of a multitude of sensory dimensions. It is involved in our experience of such things as: a chronic illness; digestive imbalance; anxiety and/or cardiovascular issues; chronic fatigue; as well as issues with cognitive function, as well as deciding what would be considered socially appropriate behavior.

Emotional attachment styles are also informed by the condition of our nervous system, and how one chooses to communicate in response to different physical and emotional stimuli. Responses to emotional stimuli, or triggers, may be responsive, or reactive and reflexive, regulated through innate neural connections, formed from biology and childhood development.

The Polyvagal complex governs our natural capacity to socially engage with others, as a function of the levels of nurturing that we received during our early years in life.

Our innate ability to self regulate our emotional state, as well as our ability to heal from inflammation and disease, are directly correlative to the health of our ANS, and the resilience of our Ventral Vagus.

One cannot view an emotional or physical condition in isolation; we are in the midst of a continual process of balance and equilibrium within our neuroendocrine system.

With the reveal of the *Polyvagal Theory*, we began to understand the human stress response in a much different way than before, and suddenly it was like a veil was lifted, and the physiology of reflexive stress responses, and human reaction to trauma, made much more sense.

No longer was there the dualistic model of stress defined only by "Sympathetic" and "Parasympathetic" states, or "fight or flight" and "rest and digest," as typically taught in traditional Western physiology; we now have another dimension of understanding that creates a *hierarchy* of organization within the Autonomic Nervous System, and explains how our bodies prioritize certain basic physiological functions during times of acute and chronic stress.

Suddenly, human responses to stress were understood with much more nuance. This understanding now includes some direction as to how our nervous system perceives stress, beyond our cognitive awareness; as well as how we self-regulate, and co-regulate with other humans, as a means to cope with stress, and rebalance our biological and emotional reflexes and reactions...

Moreover, a better understanding is now in view, of the effects of not having adequate support, and the ability to co-regulate with a trusted caregiver in the early stages of the development of our nervous system. This has lead to a much greater appreciation of the long term impacts of early childhood development on the whole body system, emotionally, energetically, and physiologically.

The *Polyvagal Theory* redefined the Autonomic Nervous System.

"Through the lens of *Polyvagal Theory*, a regulated nervous system is a nervous system that is not always in Ventral; the goal for regulation… (and regulation brings flexibility, which brings resilience)… it's about noticing that 'I leave Ventral,' and knowing that I can find my way back…

A regulated system is a system that can dysregulate and come back to regulation… A dysregulated system is a system that has these rigid response patterns, where if I get pulled out of my home in Ventral… and end up in my home away from home, in Dorsal… I can't find my way back; I'm stuck there, and for many of us that's not an uncommon experience… to feel… stuck in that <u>angry, or fearful, or anxious</u> place (that's a survival response); or in that disconnected, collapsed, disappeared place…

A regulated system [is a] nervous system that can have some flexibility when moving through survival states… coming back to that safety of connection in Ventral…"

– Deb Dana, LCSW

The Hierarchy of Autonomic Nervous System Regulation

The ANS works in service to human survival. It helps keep us Safe, and operates beyond our cognition.
"We want to Stretch our nervous system, NOT Stress our nervous system"
"Pretty much ANY diagnosis in the DSM you can map to a dysregulated nervous system"
- Deb Dana, LCSW

Parasympathetic Ventral Vagal

Regulated ANS/Ability to Connect

Connection to Self, Others, and Spirit/Source energy.
Is responsible for Healthy sense of Calm and Relaxation, and the ability to Regulate in Healthy ways in Response to Stress.
Controls Breathing and Heart Rate while in a state of Safety.
Self-Regulation is based on top of the skill of CO-Regulation.

Sympathetic

Mobilization/Action

Is survival based, and responsible for the traditional concepts of "fight or flight."
Uses a great amount of energy from the body system,
AND Controls Daily Functional/Healthy Mobilization such as:
Play
The ability to mobilize, organize, and attend to functional daily tasks;
It regulates breath rhythms and heart rhythms, toward *action*.

Sympathetic-Dorsal "Freeze or Feign (Fawn)" - "deer in headlights" - Immobilized, BUT with a Kinetic type of energy that will eventually release, when the stressor lessens, to allow enough of a sense of safety to regain mobilization. Or, in the case of "Fawn," a social behavior that is attention and approval seeking; this behavior is rooted in anxiety.

Dorsal "Freeze"- Total lack of energy, completely drained, lack of Will, inability to regain mobilization through a healthy process.

Parasympathetic Dorsal Vagal

Immobilization/Dissociation

When in an immobilization stress state of dysregulation, the nervous system has no efficient way to shift into healthy regulation.
This is a "survival" state, and is due to no efficient neurological pathways to "turn off" this primitive survival response.
Symptoms include: of a lack of energy, slowing down of Autonomic processes such as: heart rate, breathing,
lowering of blood pressure, and difficulty in cognitive processing; also possible Vasovagal symptoms, including fainting.
Indicative of Self-Abandonment.
When not in a stress/survival state, the Parasympathetic Dorsal Vagus controls our digestion and assists in cellular repair.

THE *TAN* CYCLE

THE TRANSFORMATIONAL CYCLE *OF* THE RENEWED SPIRIT AFFILIATIONS

Within various traditions of healing the body, many cultures have looked to the *Five Elements* of nature (*Wood, Fire, Earth, Metal/Air, and Water)* to inform the practice of achieving balance within the energy systems of the body. Some cultures have used only four elements: *Fire, Earth, Air, and Water*; some cultures have used the element of *'Aether'* within a *Five Element* structure. Throughout history, many different civilizations have created variations of this holographic correlation of the external environment to the internal environment, in order to understand the processes of the body, through phases of healing and transformation.

The *Tan Cycle* is interesting in that it describes the flow of *qì* through the body as having a counter-clockwise movement through the organs and meridian channels of the *Five Elements,* allowing for a lifting and supporting process of energy transformation. Through this reference tool, we are better able to identify areas of blocked energy that are preventing proper function of our Autonomic Nervous System (ANS). The structure of this cycle is specifically useful when working with people that have a history of trauma. The result of the application of this cycle, is a gentle and efficient *Way* the Sprit may align with Source energy, increasing regulation of the ANS, offering potentials for transformational healing, and preparing the internal environment for a potential quantum leap out of the trauma cycle.

The *Tan Cycle* is intended to be a reference tool that focuses on supporting and lifting each spirit affiliation within the *Five Elements*, as part of a negentropic alchemical process. Please take note of the non traditional way the spirit affiliations have been attributed through the *Tan Cycle*. I will explain these nuances in further detail within this manual.

Traditional Placements of the Spirit Affiliations Within The Classical Shēng and K'o Cycles

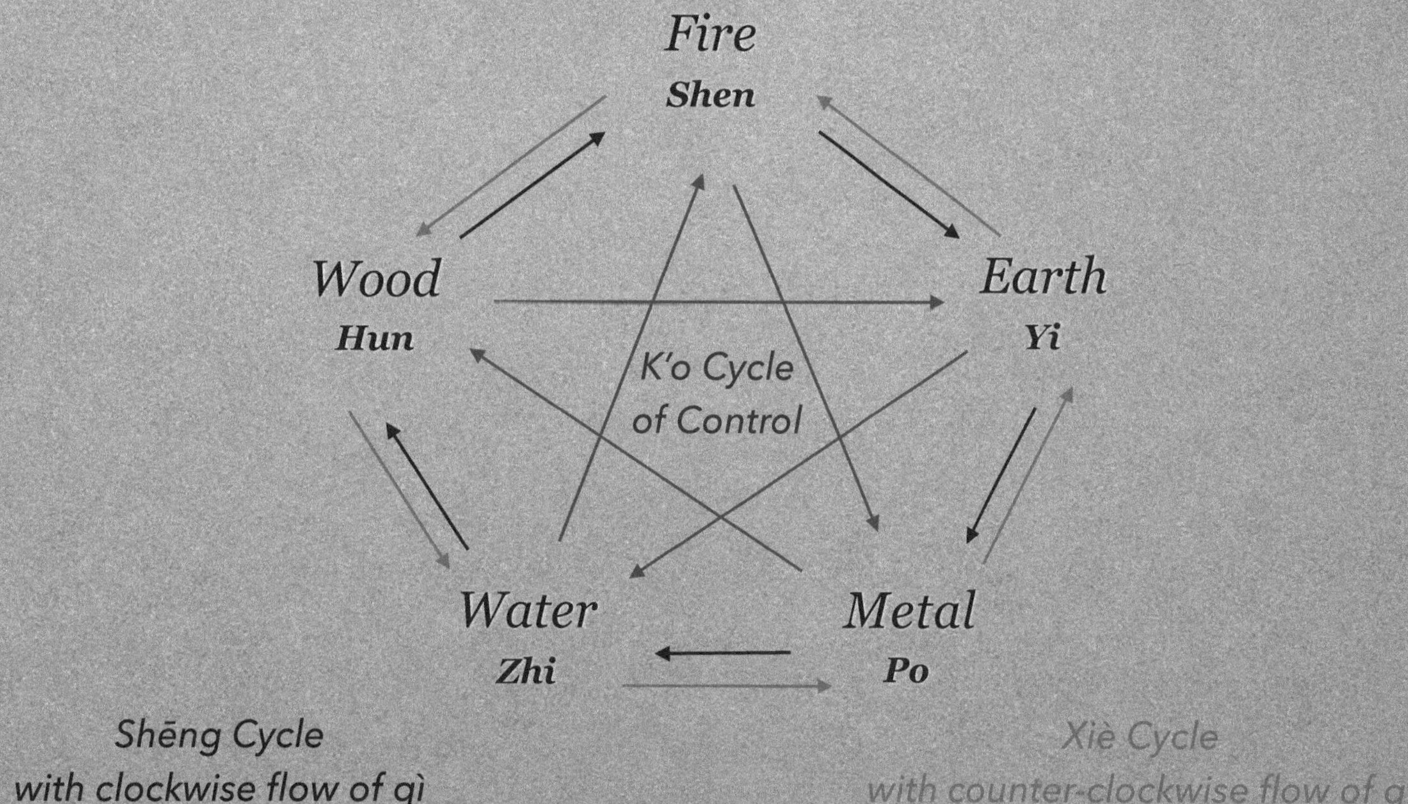

The *Tan Cycle* is not a replacement for the *Shēng Cycle*, the *Xiè Cycle*, or the *K'o Cycle*. It is an addition to those traditions, and is intended to provide a fresh perspective of the landscape of classical *Five Element* theory and traditional treatment protocol. Here, now we have a fourth reference tool that addresses the Spirit, and advances our perspective through time.

The *Tan Cycle* is based on lifting and supporting energies; whereas the *Shēng, Xiè, and K'o Cycles* of treatment are rooted in theory that is based on a philosophy of life-death-life cycles, control, destruction, and the manipulation of the environment. Inherently these ancient theories of the *Five Elements* are rooted in trauma.

Some healing traditions such as homeopathy believe in a philosophy of "like cures like"... in the case of addressing an imbalance that is due to emotional or physical trauma, I have found this not to be true... more trauma does not cure trauma, it is only more traumatizing, more toxic. Fundamentally, this energy holds us back from healing, and keeps us bound in codependent patterning.

Although the *Xiè Cycle* is also a counter-clockwise flowing cycle of treatment and evaluation, the philosophy within the clinical application, and physical movement of energy attributed to this cycle, is very different than that of the *Tan Cycle*.

The *Xiè Cycle*, as it is classically known, is in essence a trauma cycle, where the energy within the body is drained and depleted in response to traumatic physical or emotional stimulus. This cycle describes the way trauma creates pathological symptoms. These symptoms alert the observer to an imbalance within the body's innate support system.

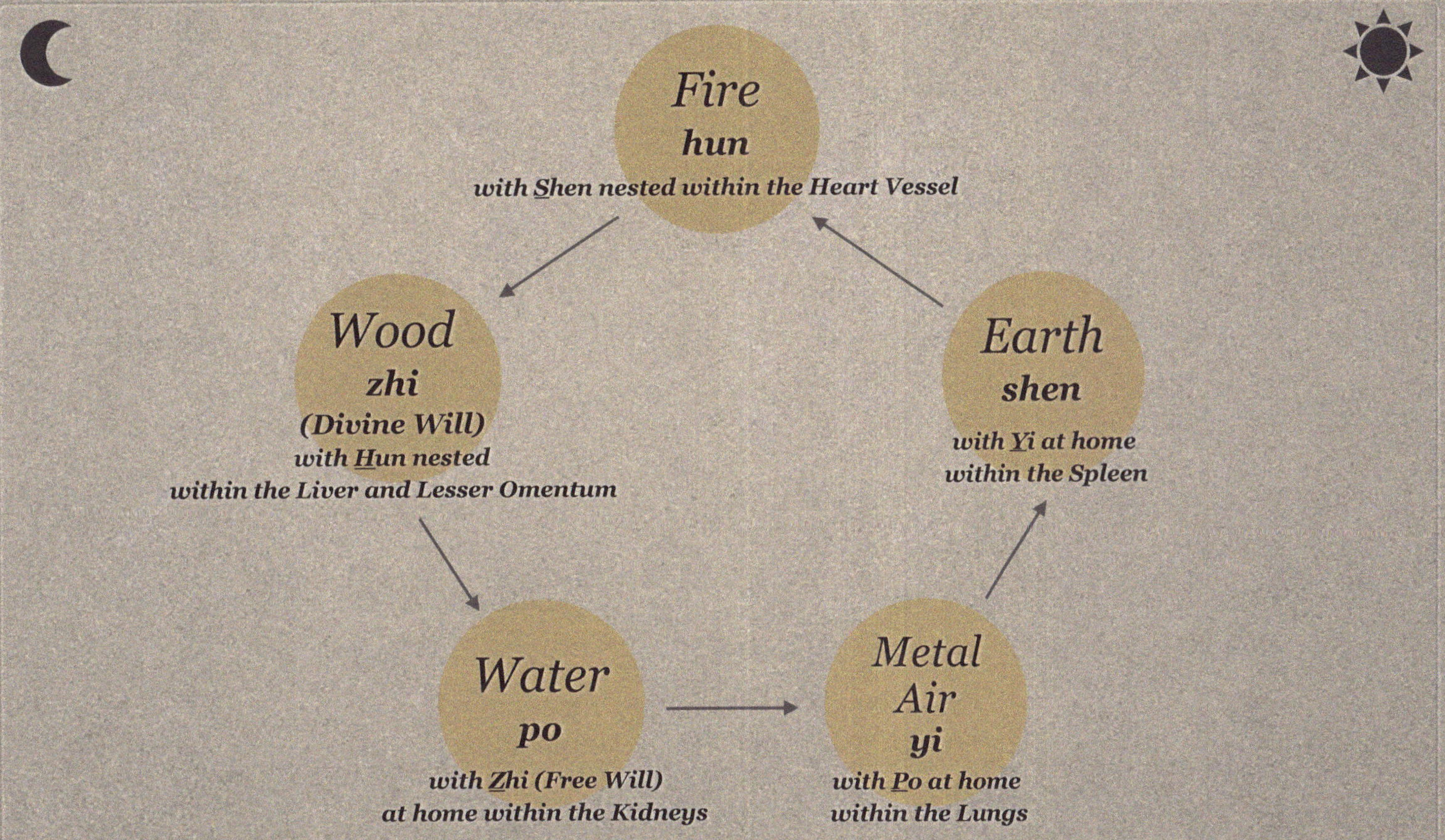

THE *TAN CYCLE*

THE *TRANSFORMATIONAL CYCLE* OF THE *RENEWED SPIRIT AFFILIATIONS*

When used as a treatment method, the movement of *qì* through the *Xiè Cycle*, by "draining," "reduction," or "exhaustion," as characterized in classical theory, is in itself inherently traumatic, and has the potential to move the flow of energy within the body further into a rhythm of dis-regulation.

By adding the *Tan Cycle* into *Five Element* treatment theory, a shift into a new perspective may be created that holds great potential for the practice of healing from trauma, providing an efficient path toward completion and transformation of traumatic cycles. I have found in my practice, that the *Tan Cycle* and the *Yu Angles,* as discussed later in this manual, have been extremely effective in assessing and healing the physiological and psychological affects of trauma within the body, achieving balance and regulation of the ANS, and healing toxic emotional response patterns.

The application of the *Tan Cycle* within *Five Element* theory, lends a harmony and ease to the treatment of clients with chronic pain and illness, complex trauma, and autoimmune conditions.

The *Tan Cycle* creates a stable structure where the spirit affiliations are advanced, into a place of protection and support, allowing for the Spirit to be welcomed into the safety of its nest, or home, within the adjacent element.

This creates a framework that is inherently holographic in nature. In this way, the energy of transformation, the *qì,* runs counter-clockwise through the cycle, allowing for the associated spirit affiliation to assist in the recovery of a Spirit that is out of balance; offering a supportive transition, and shift in energy; creating security, safety, and strength within the healing process.

This structure allows for the Observer to look past where the symptom shows up on the surface, past the psychological or physical disfunction, and into the history of the imbalance that is at the core of the layers of manifestation into disease.

The overlapping flow of the energetic spirit affiliation with the Spirit's elemental home, creates a design of a wave, similar to the *taiji* (the symbol for *yin/yang)*, and illustrative of the implied strength inherent in a Masculine energy that is lifting the Feminine energy, and a Feminine energy that is supported by a balanced and healed Masculine.

This renewal of the placements of the spirit affiliations corresponds to the progressively healed Divine Masculine *yang* energies that are rising in the Collective, along with the rise of the Divine Feminine *yin* energies, both forming into a shape that is balanced, rooted in equal appreciation.

This shift allows for the negentropic, or lifting and supporting, qualities of the healed Masculine *yang* energy to transmute, transform, and balance disharmony of the emotions and Spirits that are associated with the *yin* aspects of each element.

As we, the Collective Intelligence, progress from the Piscian age to the Age of Aquarius, naturally our spirit affiliations will shift to allow for this growth, and a confluence will form with the expanded awareness and potential for healing, permeating the Soul Collective. This happens gradually, with lifting and supportive energies, in Divine time.

Energy moves in waves; energy moves in ebb and flow.

Wood lifts and supports *Water* by the internal structure of xylem and phloem. From the Roots to the Branch, *Water* is lifted by the structure of *Wood*. Through the support and energy from the Heavens and the Sun, the warmth of the *Fire* element, calls to *Wood*, as *Wood* and *Fire* manifest this transformation of *Water* into the Sky; this is the alchemical process of transpiration.

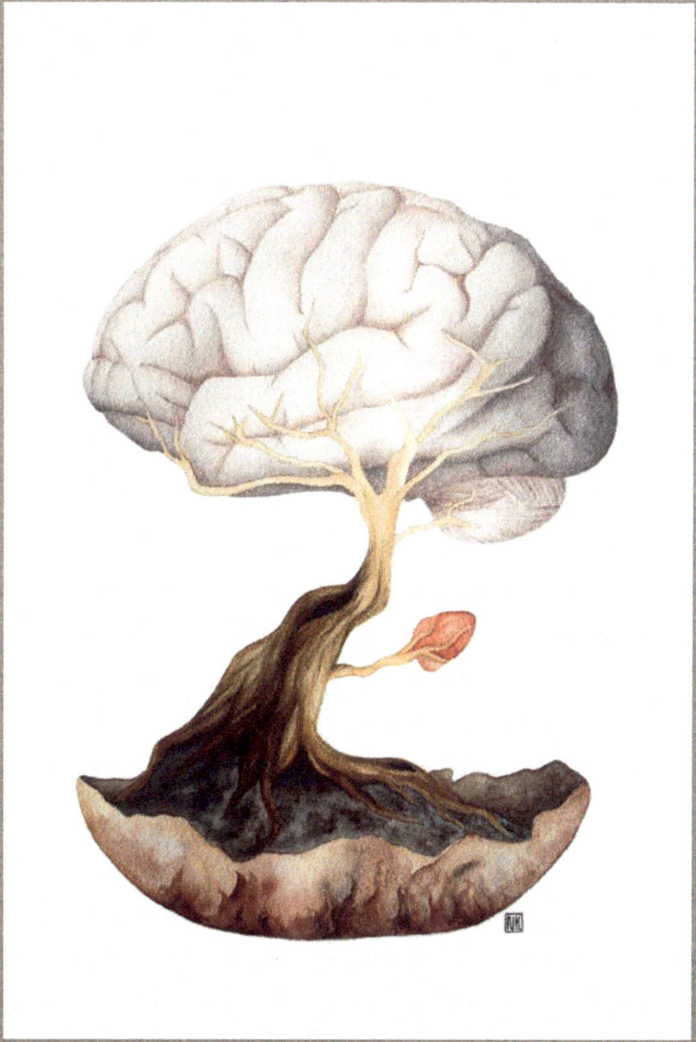

"Quercus Vagus" Watercolor © 2020 Nicole Rachelle Keane, Gratitude Healing Arts, LLC

"True Wisdom requires both Knowledge and Intuition."

- H.H. The Dalai Lama, From an address to his community in Choglamsar, Ladakh, 2011

THE CHARACTER FOR *ZHI*

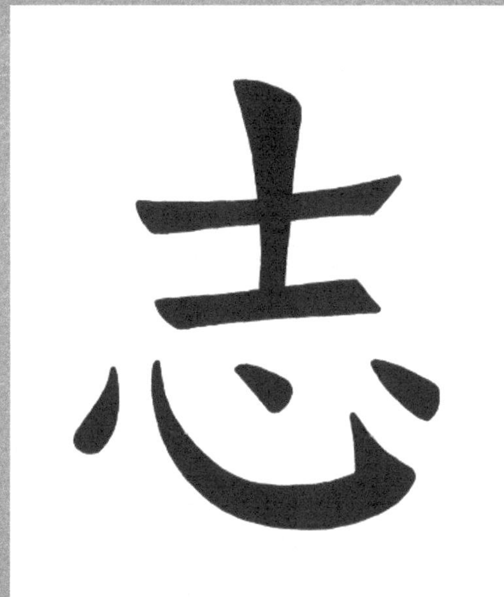

"The character for *zhi* shows us the picture of the open bowl of the heart. Above it is the radicle indicating a new green plant ascending upward from the depths of the dark earth toward the sunlight of heaven…the heart, the vessel containing the light of the [S]hen, is pictured below the upshooting sprout of the *zhi*. The hidden wisdom of this character tells us that in order to stabilize the will and achieve wisdom, the *yang* light of the [S]hen must go below the *yin*. The light of the [S]pirit becomes the root of foundation. Here, conscious awareness does not direct us from above or force the instincts or ways of nature. Rather, it lowers itself down to support our original nature as we walk through the world. The power and potency of our instincts is stabilized by the knowing of our hearts."

- Lori Eve Dachar, 'Five Spirits'

Attributes of the Wood Element

Spirit Affiliation - *zhi*

Organ officials: Liver *yin,* Gallbladder *yang*

It is my interpretation that the transformation of energies, especially in clients with a history of complex trauma, starts with the virtue of Wisdom that is inherent within the *Wood* element, as the "roots of resilience," and the spirit affiliation of *zhi.*

"The Will is responsible for the virtue of Wisdom (*zhi*). Wisdom is not certainty or knowledge. One cannot decide to obtain this Wisdom; it comes on its own. It accumulates like our years. Wisdom is a knowing that has to do with learning to have a relationship with what is unknown and unknowable. Wisdom infuses; it does not proclaim. Wisdom has some of the qualities of fear in that it has a relationship to the unknown; but unlike fear, it possesses a deep trust that the unknown eventually reveals an inevitable destiny." (*Kaptchuk*)

By working with the energy channels of the *Wood* element, one can affect the *zhi* more directly than working with the other meridians. The *zhi* spirit affiliation of the *Wood* element is the embodiment of Divine Will. The *zhi* has the ability to support, lift, transmute, and transform the Fear that is attributed to the *Water* element. Within the *Water* element, the Kidney, is the holographic domicile of the *Zhi* Spirit. This is the seat of the Free Will, or the human desires of the Ego self, from which much Fear arises. Just as the xylem within a tree raises water toward the light, eventually realizing vapor into the atmosphere through the alchemical process of transpiration, the *Wood* element transmutes the energy within *Water* to the sky, aligning the Corporeal Soul and *jing* with the heavens, guided on the path of Divine Will and intrinsic Wisdom.

The *zhi*, in its highest manifestations, corresponds to being in a state of Ventral Vagal regulation. When the *zhi* is not strong enough to lift and support the Kidneys, due to energetic or physical restrictions within the Liver or Gallbladder meridians, the body responds to emotional and environmental stressors with Fear and Sympathetic activation.

The emotion of the Kidney out of balance is Fear. "Fear detects the unknown, but it has the same energetic quality that is sensitive to, and can embrace, Wisdom and the trust of faith. The [Divine] Will transmutes angst into Wisdom." *Id*.

Therefore, it is the *zhi*, spirit affiliation of the *Wood* element, that supports and lifts the Spirit of the *Water* element in disharmony, the *Zhi* that rests within the Kidney.

By working physically and energetically within the meridian of the *yang* organ of the *Wood* element, the Gallbladder, one can offer transformational support and lifting energy to imbalance and disharmony within the *yin* organ of the *Water* element, the Kidney. This support from the Gallbladder is directed by the corresponding *yin* organ, the Liver, also known in classical Asian medical theory as "the General of the Army."

This is an example of how the negentropic effect of the healed Masculine *yang* energy works together with assistance from the deeper levels of *yin* energy within the elements. Through alignment with the *zhi*, the Divine Will, a pathway is created to supportive and transformational healing of the *Water* element, as illustrated within the counterclockwise flow of *qì* through the *Tan Cycle*. A balance in the dance between *yin* and *yang*, *zhi* supporting *Zhi;* a healing potential created by the flow between the Soul and the Self, in supportive resonance and lifting harmony.

In the case of disfunction within the energetic or physical structure of the *yang* organ of the *Water* element, the Bladder, the Observer would look first toward disfunction within the *yin* channels of the same element, the Kidney, for any restrictions that may be creating a distortion in physical structure, or an imbalance of energy flow.

Once the *yin* elemental counterpart has been consulted, then the Observer would look toward the lifting and supporting nature of the organs of the *Wood* element, meridians, and channel divergencies for treatment potentials, as described. This method of assessment of the flow of energy, or *qì*, is Universally applicable throughout the *Tan Cycle*.

Disfunction within the *Wood* element may manifest in metabolic and energetic lethargy, or excess, as well as Anger and irritation. "A weak *yang* Will means profound passivity and being devoid of assertiveness. A deficiency of the *yin* Will may produce such signs as the absence of tranquility, or deep restlessness. A diminished *yin* Will may also cause the *yang* Will to become reckless and unrestrained…Inordinate existential fear can result from Will disturbances." *Id.*

Such is indicative of an inability to *receive* and *implement* the guidance of the higher Self, and a lack of awareness of one's innate potentials. This is a result of a breakdown of the *Tan Cycle,* with deficiency of *Wood* stemming from physical or energetic restrictions within *Fire* and *Earth*.

This "inordinate existential fear," that is spoken of previously, is associated with the Kidneys, and is a product of the *zhi,* the Divine Will of the *Wood* element, being unable to support and lift the *Zhi* Spirit, or Free Will, that is home within the *Water* element. Free Will associated with the concept known as the human Ego. *Wood* is weak because it is not adequately supported by the energy of *Earth* and *Fire;* this is a level of self abandonment and lack of trust in the Self.

If left unsupported by the *Wood* element, the Fear associated with the *Water* element will manifest in Sympathetic Nervous System (SNS) stress activation, commonly characterized by the "fight or flight" spectrum of behavior.

Anatomically, this response involving the SNS is mediated by the Ventral Vagus, and is a function of the hierarchical organization of the nervous system, which is physiologically more related to the health of the *Wood* element, the *Fire* element, and the *Earth* element, than that of the *Water* element, due to the Ventral and Dorsal Vagal afferent pathways being governors of the Autonomic Nervous System (ANS).

The inherent Vagal tone, or the general health of the ANS within an individual, helps to determine the potential reserves of resilience that one may access when in stressful situations.

Vagal tone, and the general health of the ANS, is a function of various aspects of allostatic load within an individual, related to impacts such as: the microbial balance of the viscera, viral load, toxin load, emotional stressors, and trauma history. Energetically, this attribute is "Governed" by the Liver, the General.

By referencing the *Tan Cycle*, treatment plans for symptoms associated with the *Water* element, may involve the *Wood* element, as well as the *Fire* element. These elements function to lift and support the Spirit disharmony of the Free Will of the *Zhi*, seated in the Kidney. The Ventral Vagal regulation of the *Wood* and *Fire* elements help transform the trauma and stress response characteristic of Sympathetic activation.

Treatment of the organs and pathways associated with the *Wood* element may have a prolific effect on the Polyvagal complex, and have ripple effects throughout the rest of the elements, due to the flow of *qì*, through the *Tan Cycle,* lifting and supporting the *Water* and *Metal/Air* elements, as well as the reach that these energy channels have throughout the body, specifically the Bladder, and the nexus between the peripheral nervous system, Sympathetic activation, and systemic inflammation.

When the *zhi* of the *Wood* element is disturbed, and not strong enough to support and lift the *Water* element, manifestations may include:

- extreme exhaustion,
- lack of initiative,
- reduced short term memory,
- challenges recollecting recent events,
- insomnia from agitation,
- high blood pressure,
- anxiety,
- chronic fatigue,
- inability to *respond* instead of *react;* and
- what is typical of a "short fuse," characteristic of annoyance and stress response.

These symptoms are indicative of a breakdown in the ability of the *yang* aspects of the Gallbladder and Liver to support and lift the *yin* functions of the Kidney and Adrenal, such as receptivity and playfulness, the positive side of the Sympathetic Nervous System (SNS).

The *zhi* of the *Wood* element, and the ANS governance of the stress response, is linked to the Kidney meridian and the Adrenal glands, through the Hypothalamus, Pituitary, Adrenal axis (HPA axis), and SNS response to Fear, a "fight or flight" reaction initiated by the Neuroendocrine system.

Extreme imbalance of the *Wood* element, and the spirit of *zhi,* can also result in the "freeze or feign" spectrum of symptoms associated with Parasympathetic Dorsal Vagal domination of the stress response. This spectrum of reaction shuts down connection to Divine Will, and disables Free Will. This will be discussed in more detail in subsequent chapters, as a "backsliding" within the *Tan Cycle.*

In chronic cases, Dorsal Vagal dominance may disable healthy digestion through energetic irregularities in the *afferent* and *efferent* Vagal pathways that involve the Nodose Ganglion in the Hepatic Hilum, and the Vagal Nuclei in the Medulla.

"Healing the *zhi* must include listening to the voices of the *po.*" (*Dachar)*

In the *Tan Cycle*, the *po* is associated with the *Water* element. As part of the *Tan Cycle* treatment theory, the Observer would listen to the symptoms that are out of balance within the *Water* element, and then listen for energetic or physical restrictions within the Liver or Gallbladder meridians, and collateral divergent channels, for a "cause."

After restrictions are released within the *Wood* element, the flow of *qì* through the *Tan Cycle* may empower the body to transmit the lifting and supporting energy of *Wood* to the *Water* element, initiating renewal. The elements at *Yu Angles* from the symptoms in question can also be assessed to assist in restoration of the flow of *qì,* this will be discussed in later chapters as well.

The *zhi* can be especially effected by emotional and environmental toxicity. The Liver is the organ responsible for cleansing the blood of toxins, and filters out toxicity as efficiently as it is able. Moreover, the nervous system, and process of myelination, is significantly affected by the presence of toxins such as chemicals, allergens, and heavy metals. These contaminants both collect within Cranial nuclei and higher order neurons, and contribute to reduction in essential vitamins, amino acids, and minerals, that are exhausted through the process of detoxification and methylation by the Liver.

Potential sources of emotional toxicity that contribute to physiological disfunction include a person being exposed to behaviors within significant relationships such as:

- passive aggressiveness,
- narcissistic behavior,
- neglect, and
- physical or emotional abuse.

Environmental toxicity sources include:

- molds,
- cleaning products,
- paints and paint thinners,
- solvents, and
- fumes from fuels.

In addition to affecting the capacity for emotional regulation, significant or chronic toxicity issues can also inhibit the body's ability to digest and assimilate proteins and fats. This is due to the interference of toxins within the *afferent* and *efferent* neural network of the ANS, potentially affecting the chemical processes associated with digestion.

Many of the neural structures that are affected by toxicity are located within the main Gallbladder meridian, and Divergent channel, including areas of the Polyvagal complex.

Often times Thyroid disfunction, hypo or hyper, will be accompanied by disfunction in the Gallbladder, as the Thyroid is within the Gallbladder Divergent channel.

There may also be a physical restriction in or around the Gallbladder itself that is contributing to the disruption in the flow of energy through the channels, potentially affecting distant places within the landscape of the body.

A short memory, and the inability to retain and recall information, may also be a sign that emotional toxicity, trauma, or stress is affecting the *Wood* element, and creating a disturbance of the *zhi*.

The information processing and storage functions of the Hippocampus, Amygdala, and Temporal lobe, are affected by stress and blockages within the Gallbladder meridian, as this energy channel runs along the temporal aspect of the Cranium, connecting with these inter-Cranial structures and nuclei.

The anatomical relationships of the structures associated with the *Wood* and *Earth* elements, are very related to the spectrum of Parasympathetic Dorsal Vagal response to stressors, due to their placement below the Diaphragm, and their energetic affiliations to aspects of Self perception, as well as how one is perceived by Others. The Lesser Omentum, of the Triple Warmer channel within the *Fire* element, is also associated with this relationship, as it provides the connective tissue and ligamentous support within this specific area.

"The light of self-awareness [self worth] is crucial for the healthy functioning of the *zhi*. Without this light, the *zhi* is like a plant that does not receive adequate sunlight. Its growth will be stunted, or the plant will shoot up wildly searching for light but there will be no strength in its roots." (*Dachar, Five Spirits*)

If the sense of Self is not able to be accessed because it is being, or was in the past, repressed in some way energetically, then social engagement behaviors may become distorted and lead to isolation behaviors. If the Self of the individual was never adequately nurtured and supported as a child, an individual may experience challenges which can include becoming overly self focused, or at times dissociated, in order to compensate for neglect, emotional abuse, or physical trauma.

The "shame, guilt, and fear" triad that is a hallmark of the Narcissistic behavior spectrum is especially prevalent in disturbances of the *zhi*, and the *Wood* element, as well as the spirit affiliation for the *Earth* element, due to a deep inability to identify with a healthy sense of Self.

Moreover, often clients that exhibit a spectrum of these behavior traits, also have significant physical restrictions of the Liver and the Stomach relative to the Diaphragm, or physiological disfunction of the Liver, Gallbladder, Stomach, and Spleen/Pancreas.
The psychosocial manifestations of this energy block include:

- manipulation,
- lying,
- dissociation,
- lack of empathy, and
- extreme need for control in various areas of life.

This energetic block associated with disturbance of the *Wood* element and the *Earth* element, is a pathology involving the dominance of the Dorsal Vagal complex, and can be triggered to greater or lesser extent by neuroceptive cues that initiate a survival response.

To heal from this significant spectrum of disharmony requires a reorganizing of the nervous system, and intimate work supporting the Spirit of the *Wood* element. This is done through working with the spirit affiliations within the *Tan Cycle,* and following guidance for release of physical and energetic restrictions through indirect techniques that work with the *Earth* and *Metal/Air* elements, as suggested by the *Yu Angles.*

A healing of this order requires surrender and alignment with *zhi,* or Divine Will, through spirit affiliation guidance of the *hun* of the *Fire* element, and the light of the *Shen* within the Heart, as well as support from the *shen,* affiliated with the Earth element, and a healthy *Yi* within the Spleen, that is supported by the holographic reflection of the *yi* within the *Metal* element.

The empowering energies that result from finding one's purpose through alignment with Source light foster a strong sense of self identity. This allows the Spirit to root down within, and is essential in healing and empowering the *zhi,* returning Wisdom and balance to the Divine Will.

To return to a path of unhindered, unconditional acceptance and appreciation, requires unbiased Wonder about what the future holds, while retaining the Wisdom gained through experience; this is the highest manifestation of the *zhi.*

This healed space is essential in order to effectively carry out the attributes of Instinctual Power, the alignment of Divine Will with Free Will, and the embodiment of Courage.

"The closest Western word for the Chinese sense of Wisdom is probably faith. This faith does not imply a parochial religious identity, but speaks to a sense of trust and being able to embrace the unknown."

– Ted Kaptchuk, 'The Web That Has No Weaver'

Embracing Faith Through *zhi*

The Wisdom of Faith is the ability to respond instead of react, to trust in a Divine path, and to actualize the ease with which the *Tao* unfolds.

When in balance and functioning optimally, the *Wood* and *Water* elements provide the harmony for the presence of Divine Will to be manifest by Free Will on the Earth plane.

Lori Eve Dechar in her book "Five Spirits" says, "the realm of the zhi spirits is the realm of what Vedic philosophers called karma, the realm of the unconscious forces and collective energy threads that determine the course of our lives."

I read this as a description of the trauma cycle that plays out within some lives, to greater or lesser degree, depending on one's heritage and innate resilience; as well as the effect that this trauma has on one's psyche and Autonomic Nervous System (ANS).

As described within the *Polyvagal Theory*, the human nervous system is organized in such a way that the body perceives trauma and stress in certain degrees, specific to each person. This quality of resilience, and level of inherent "Wisdom" within the nervous system, determines the course of our lives, from a physiological, as well as psychological perspective.

We can cultivate the Wisdom of faith through the trust that unfolds as we gain more awareness of how, and why, our nervous system reacts to the trauma and stress that we experience.

The Resilience of *zhi*

The Divine Will, or *zhi* spirit, is the "root of resilience," with the virtue of Wisdom, that is gained from experience; it is the spirit of the *Wood* element.

The Psychological functions of the *zhi* are:

- Instinctual Power, and
- Aligned Divine Will and Courage, like a Warrior or General, with a knowing of exactly how to strategize for an advance, and swiftly respond effectively to any attack.

Psychospiritual challenges of the *zhi* are:

- Surrendering to the Tao, or releasing the need for control,
- Allowing life to just *Be*, as well as
- Returning to Origin, or allowing the mind to arise from a state of *pu*, the "uncarved block."

This State of being, *pu,* is related to the ability to be resilient, having an innate or acquired buffer to the traumas and dramas of life that color and shape our present and future experiences.

We may find enjoyment in connection, and greater empathy for society as a whole, as the benevolence imparted by the virtues of the *Fire* element, and the *hun,* illuminates the energy of the *Wood* element, easing the growth and development of equanimity. Once we are able to feel stable within ourselves, trusting our inner senses, we are able to approach life without bias, be less reactive, and more in a state of perpetual Gratitude and Wonder.

This positive feedback loop, initiated within the *Five Element* system, through the balancing, lifting, and supporting energies of the *Tan Cycle*, begins with physical and energetic balance of the *Wood* element.

Through relation to the supporting and lifting aspects of the *Fire* element, and the *Earth* element, this creation process enables a safe space, which allows for alchemical transformation.

As the *zhi* begins to balance and heal through empowering the *Wood* element, the ANS will begin to shift toward a more secure place, able to self regulate within the Parasympathetic Ventral Vagal state more easily.

Our physiology and psychology are more secure; our branches being blown less wildly in the winds of life.

This happens through the warmth of the lifting and supporting aspects of the *Fire* element, and is aided, in great respect, by the process of co-regulation and the Social Engagement System.

The energetic, anatomical, and physiological links between the *Wood - Fire - Earth* pathways, accessed within the *Tan Cycle,* lay the foundation for Autonomic regulation and resiliency through the Polyvagal system.

When the *Wood - Fire - Earth* pathway is in harmony, Ventral Vagal regulation during times of stress or trauma is more accessible to us, and our bodies have less irritation, inflammation, and physical and emotional pain, universally.

To receive the insight and intuition essential to heal the *zhi* of the *Wood* element, the Soul requires the guidance and light of the *hun* and the *shen* of the *Fire* and the *Earth* elements, and the pure illumination of a vibrant *Shen*, nested within the *Heart*. Aspects that are characteristic of this process include:

- the renewal of an excitement for life, and identification of personal passions or interests;
- greater trust in one's Self, intuitions, and a sense of acceptance of "Diving Timing;"
- empowered balance within emotional responses, and the ability to learn and grow through challenging experiences;
- the ability to pursue potential futures with a wonder of possibility, as opposed to the anxiety of the unknown;
- a sense of non-Egoic pride and Integrity; greater self acceptance;
- equanimity with regard to one's external environment, no longer prioritizing a need for control; and
- a greater "trust in the process," and ability to have "faith."

As our ANS becomes well balanced and resilient, we are able to connect with our internal Self, reflect, and grow; we are able to identify how we feel, and express ourSelves appropriately, connecting in healthy ways with our environment.

The chakra associated with the *zhi* spirit and the *Wood* element is the Throat chakra, corresponding to the Pharyngeal plexus; balance and alignment of this energy center allows for the ability to "speak our truth," and to be in touch with the grace of that internal knowing.

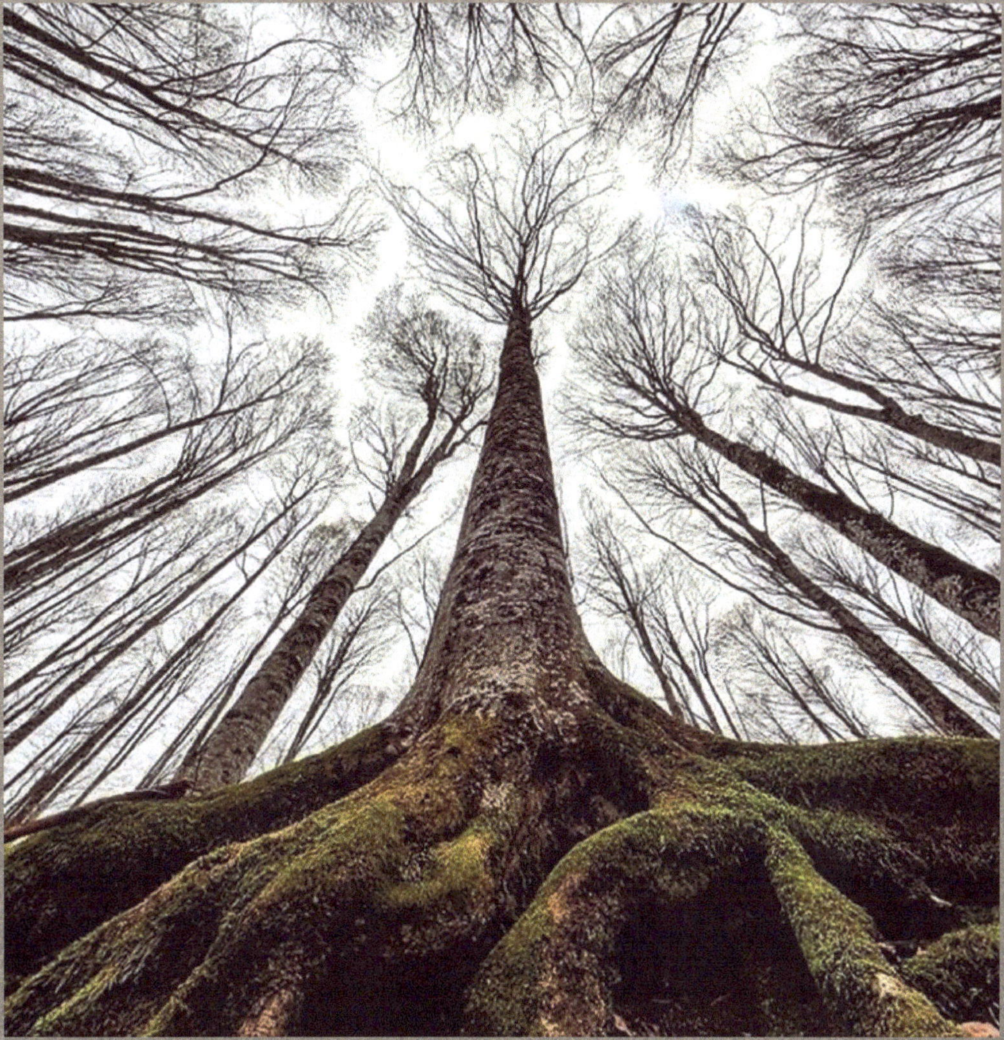

© Carletto Del Monaco

The *Fire* element lifts and supports the *Wood* element by providing the heat, or energy, that *Wood,* which is symbolic of life in general, needs to grow and flourish. The energy of our solar *Fire,* the Sun, is essential for the *Wood* element to call on *Water,* for growth, and the *Minerals* of the *Earth* for nourishment.

The energy of *Fire,* through the warmth of the Heart, transforms life, and sustains and supports processes of transition. From seed to plant, and eventually back to the Earth from where it came, by the magic of the flame, life renews through growth and transformation.

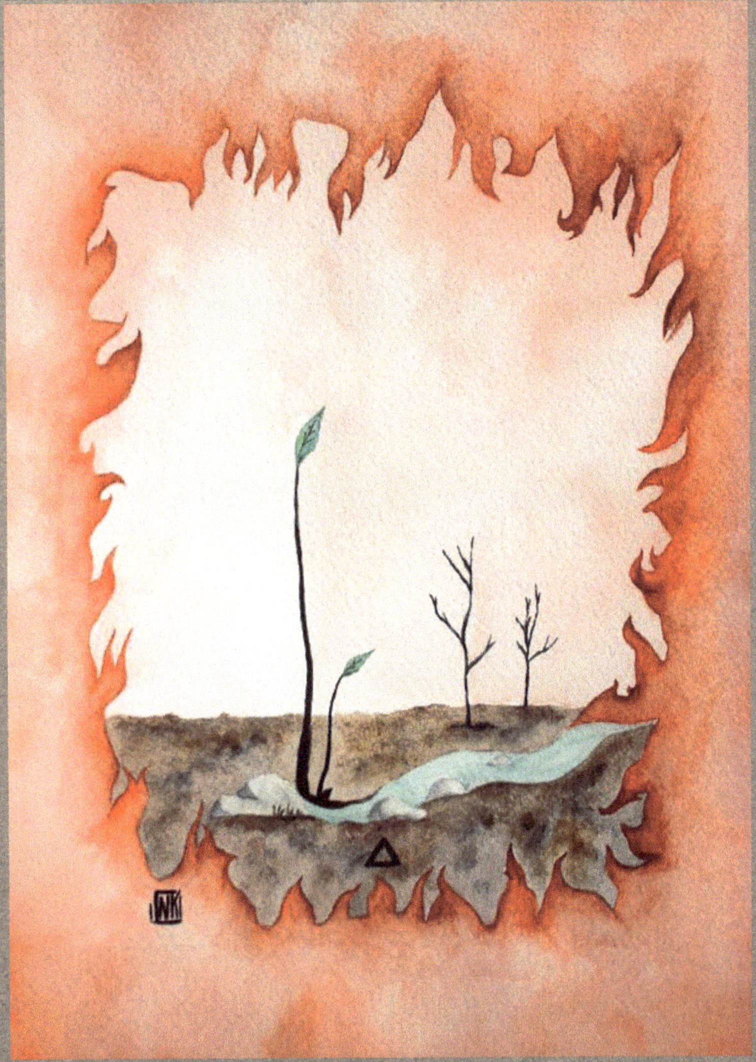

"Renewal," Watercolor © 2020 Nicole Rachelle Keane, Gratitude Healing Arts, LLC

"Bodhichitta is sometimes compared to the sun; our patterns of putting up barriers are like clouds that cover it. Like the sun, bodhichitta is always shining, so as the clouds begin to dissolve, our true nature shines through…openness of heart and mind is always available to us - right here, right now - even when we feel hopelessly shut-down.

To uncover it, all we need is gentleness, kindness - and patience."

- Pema Chodron, 'Tonglen: The Path of Transformation'

THE CHARACTER FOR *HUN*

魂

"The character for *hun* is made up of a combination of the radical for *yun* (clouds) and the radical for *gui* [disembodied spirit or ghost]. It reminds us that the *hun* are related to the breaths and to the spirits, and that the *hun*...are free to come and go...Like the clouds, the hun cannot be pinned down. Yet also like the clouds, they are influenced by the vicissitudes of life on the material plane...the light of the *hun* is partially dependent on the nourishment of the earth. It must be fed by matter, in order for it to shine...the *hun* are the agents of penetration who bring the spiritual resonances of the *shen* down to the earth so that they can enter into form, space, and time."

-Lori Eve Dachar, 'Five Spirits'

Attributes of the Fire Element

Spirit Affiliation - *hun*

Organ officials: Triple Warmer *yang,* Small Intestine *yin;* Pericardium *yang,* Heart *yin*

The concept of *hun,* as a spirit affiliation, is a bit ethereal. It is described as the "Non-Corporeal Soul," or the aspect of one's essence that is not bound to the body in the physical realm. It may function as a wayshower, like a flock of birds signaling the turning of a season; they connect the physical body with gentle direction and guidance from another realm. The *hun* provide a direct connection with the Oversoul, or Collective Unconscious, and can be affected by both benefic and malefic influences and energies from other realms. The *hun* have qualities of both a flock of birds, and the smoke from a fire seen settling in a valley, or drifting up and away with the wind.

"The *hun* is considered part of the person that is 'not attached to the physical body' and supposedly continues to exist after the cessation of life." (*Kaptchuk*)

In this way, the *hun* may be the spiritual mechanism through which trauma patterns are passed down through generations; in some cases, creating epigenetic changes to physical and emotional patterns within a family lineage. This could be due to an energetic nexus between the *hun* and the Kidneys of the Water Element, should the individual not align with the Divine guidance and support given within a lifetime, from the *hun* and the *zhi*.

Just as the *hun* are likened to a flock of birds when the body is in the physical form, they are much like the unlimited sparks of a bonfire in the presence of death. With each small death that we experience in human form, the *hun* guide our Soul's direction on the paths of transformations that we follow through this lifetime. Like a Phoenix rising from the flames; the *hun* are both the Phoenix and the flames; they are what guides us, with courage, into the fire. To transform, one first has to go within, and allow for an aspect of Self to be purified through the transformation of the flame.

In their highest manifestations, the flames of the *hun* transcend dimensions and alchemize organic, dark matter, or emotion, into the smoke that drifts like clouds through the valleys, waiting for the winds of change and integration.

Cultures throughout history have used fire, in ceremony, to both release the body from, and return the body to, the Earth realm, alchemizing the Soul. As such, the spirit affiliation of the *Fire* element in the *Tan Cycle* is the *hun*.

The *Hun* Spirit require a safe place to nest, as they motion between the physical and the Spirit world. When *Hun* are able to come and go from a place of safety, there is an intrinsic support that is present. This sense of safety to roam, allows the *Hun* Spirit to receive an awareness of the 'the Other' that is essential to the cultivation and expression of appropriate levels of empathy toward our immediate surroundings, and greater community, that we exist within.

The *Hun* are able to provide an awareness of suffering, outside of the Self, from the experiences of different energies they collect during their flights about the world at large; just as they bring back to the nest an awareness of lives lived, they bring also an appreciation for a world that is in balance. They can then radiate this spectrum of knowing, from the safety of a supported nest within the body that they occupy in this lifetime, this awareness takes on the form of *Gratitude*.

"When we are in a state of *gratitude*, we are bathed in cues of safety," Dr. Stephen Porges.

When the *Hun* are unable to return to a place of safety within the body, or have been so affected by their experience of suffering along their travels, that they are unable to leave the body evermore, the subconscious emotional burden that this captive situation creates often manifests in imbalance and disease within the Autonomic Nervous System (ANS).

Under these conditions, the *hun* spirit affiliated with the *Fire* element is no longer able to lift and support the *Wood* element, and the nervous system is unable to access sustainable pathways for Parasympathetic Ventral Vagal regulation.

In the physical body, the Spirit *Hun* is aligned with the tissue system and energy channels of the Triple Warmer, within the *Fire* element. The *Hun* are considered predominantly *yang* in nature, just as the Triple Warmer. As the concept of *hun*, as a spirit affiliation, is a bit ephemeral, as the "Non-Corporeal Soul," so too are the physical aspects of the Triple Warmer.

I have seen the Triple Warmer described as the three energy centers, or *dantian;* I have heard it referred to as the energetic description of the Lymphatic system; as well as a number of other curious and contemplative suggestions.

In my clinical practice, I have observed the Triple Warmer, in direct relation to the Spirit of *Hun*, as three areas of the body that are specifically associated with deposits of Brown Adipose Tissue (BAT): the Thoracic Inlet, or Superior Thoracic Aperture (the Supraclavicular area); the Lesser Omentum; and the Greater Omentum. BAT atrophies with age in most humans, and is stored in other areas of the body, including the areas surrounding the Thymus, Kidneys, and upper back.

Specifically, I have noticed that most often in cases of trauma history, the Spirit *Hun,* the holographic representation of *hun* in the physical body, make their presence known by nesting in the Biliary Tree, within the Lesser Omentum, close to the *yin* Liver. This location supports a special relationship which intricately links energetic aspects of the *Wood* element and *Fire* element, that support the healthy regulatory functioning of the Parasympathetic Ventral Vagal complex, by assisting the Dorsal Vagus with balance and integration when in proper function.

Perhaps this is why the *hun* spirit affiliation has been traditionally attributed to the Liver of the *Wood* element, as the Lesser Omentum is physically connected to the Liver, and in fact provides a ligamentous, fascial, and lymphatic, bridge of connective tissue between the Stomach and the Liver.

When the Spirit *Hun* are at home, nesting, within the Lesser Omentum, they are able to connect the *shen* of the *Earth* element, to the *zhi* of the *Wood* element; by inhabiting a physical and energetic pathway of lifting and supporting energies within the *Tan Cycle,* and as long as they are able to fly through the pathways of the *Fire* element, they may provide a direct link between Spirit source energy and the human body.

Where there is no feeling of a "safe nest" to come home to, within the Lesser Omentum, the body may descend into chaotic vibration, due to the inability of the Ventral Vagus to effectively regulate emotional stability and inflammation processes. Symptoms of this *Hun* disturbance may include:

- dissociation,
- depression or creative block,
- sleepless nights over worry or anxiety regarding relationships or decisions involving communication,
- increased inflammation and pain,
- lack of vocal prosody, or intonation and variation in vocal pitch;
- ANS dysregulation, and
- chronic or autoimmune illness.

In cases of extreme disturbance of the *hun spirit affiliation*, as well as the *Shen* that nest in the Heart, and the *shen* that are affiliated with the *Earth* element, a person may experience symptoms of a personality that is disordered.

The inability of the *hun* of the *Fire* element to lift and support the *zhi* of the *Wood* element within the regenerative alchemical burning process, results in a kind of bedlam. After all, a successful General, the Liver, must have good advisors… Where there is no sense of perspective afforded by the *hun*, the function of the Liver and the Gallbladder, as well as the other organs and structures along their corresponding energy channels, will suffer.

When the *hun* are not able to fulfill their supportive role within the *Tan* Cycle, the *Wood* element is unable to function with ease, and the Parasympathetic Ventral Vagal nervous system is not able to appropriately process and integrate exposure to stress and trauma.

This causes the Sympathetic stress response, governed by the *po*, affiliated with the *Water* element, to rise like a wave in attempts to manage and control situations, often creating more chaos. And if the *po* becomes too disrupted, the pool of water becomes a well of stagnation, leading into the depths of the Parasympathetic Dorsal Vagal immobilization response.

The influence of the *hun* in decision making and judgement, rests with the affiliation of the Greater Omentum (*yang*) to the Small Intestine, the *yin* paired organ to the predominantly *yang* Triple Warmer. The Small Intestine is the organ that sorts and absorbs; physically this refers to nutrients from our food sources; energetically, the sorting of good and bad attributes of a person or situation, is an essential part in the decision making process.

Moreover, an essential function of the Small Intestine is the absorption of the Wisdom gained from experiences, and the ability to actualizing that to knowing when making decisions.

Just as the *yin* Small Intestine is paired with the *yang* Triple Warmer within the description of the *Fire* element of the *Tan Cycle,* the *yin* Heart is paired with the *yang* Pericardium.

In her book, *Five Spirits,* Lori Eve Dachar describes the classical literature as stating that the *hun* reside in the eyes by day "where they help us to see and think clearly, to make wise decisions, and to direct our actions in a way that is best for our Soul's purpose;" and that "by night, the windy *hun* descend downward, sinking to the fleshy organ of the Liver where they are weighed down by the *yin* essences of the blood. At night, while we sleep, the *hun* actively organize our dreams and imagine our plans for the future."

This sounds a lot like the "rest and digest" function of the Parasympathetic Nervous System, and the beneficial effects of balanced and healthy Dorsal Vagal function. When balanced by a healthy Parasympathetic Ventral Vagal nervous system, the Dorsal Vagus is able to carry out essential functions of renewal within the internal ecosystem during our times of rest.

I find it particularly intriguing that the Small Intestine, and the Triple Warmer meridian channels, both have internal pathways that connect to the inner and outer corner of the eyes, respectively; as well as pathways that descend internally, through the areas of the Thoracic Inlet, Supraclavicular area, Lesser Omentum, and Greater Omentum. This only furthers a suggestion for the reinterpretation of the classical literature to align with the principles illustrated within the *Tan Cycle,* presented in this manual, and modern knowledge of anatomy and physiology.

The main avenues of the Social Engagement System, as described within the Polyvagal Theory, are the eyes and the muscles associated with making eye contact and facial expressions.

The Cranial nerves that govern eye contact and facial expressions connect energetically with the Triple Warmer and Small Intestine Meridians, and make anatomical and physiological connections through the Vagal Nuclei in the Brainstem, to the myelinated neurons of the Ventral Vagus, that help regulate the Heart. This suggests that the *Fire* element, and attributes of the *hun*, give rise to the Social Engagement System.

When the *hun* do not have the appropriate emotional resources during the early developmental stages of life, they do not receive proper attunement. This period of development is between two months before birth, to approximately seven to eight years of age.

It is during this time that a child is most vulnerable to the damaging effects of neglect, emotionally toxic behavior, and physical abuse.

These crucial years form the foundation of our Social Engagement System. That foundation is built by the degree of connection with a primary caregiver: the mirror and guide through which the child experiences the world. If a consistent primary caregiver is absent, or abusive, the Social Engagement System, and Autonomic Nervous System, may not develop optimally. Of course, this occurs to various degrees, depending on the situation.

In the case of a stable, supportive, loving early family life, the *hun* are able to develop in healthy ways; they leave the nest and travel along their flight path, in gradually greater and greater capacity, because they know they have the support of a loving home, to which they may return.

In cases where the early family life, is chaotic, neglectful, or abusive, the *hun* may learn to leave the nest of the *Fire* element, afraid to come back home, effectively abandoning the *Self.* This has a strong affect on the Spirit *Hun,* and may potentially lead to patterns of behavior such as:

- repetitive cycles of abusive decision making as an adult, toward the Self or others;
- difficulty in making decisions;
- self-sabotaging behaviors;
- addictions and substance abuse;
- lack of healthy boundaries in relationships;
- a pervasive sense of shame;
- inability to empathize with others;
- unpredictable and disorganized attachment styles;
- inappropriate emotional responses to interpersonal situations and communications;
- a sense that the Soul is consistently out of the body, or not being able to feel a connection with the physical self; and
- lack of self love, and consistently making choices that put oneself in the path of hardship.

Another result of trauma in early childhood, or acute emotional or physical trauma or stress that happens later in life, is when the *hun* become stuck in the body, unable to leave, unable to gain guidance from Source and experience their world in healthy ways.

When the *hun* become stuck in the body, this often manifests as the "freeze or feign/fawn" dynamic that is a function of what I call in my clinic "*hun* stuck in the chimney." This is when the *hun* are energetically unable to move within the body along the path of the Triple Warmer.

I imagine the bowels of a chimney, where all the main burning is going on, as the Greater Omentum of the Triple Warmer, the organ that covers the Small Intestines. The Lesser Omentum of the Triple Warmer, is the main chimney stack, and the upper section of the Triple Warmer, the area of the Thoracic Inlet and Supraclavicular area, is like the exit of the chimney stack.

I often see *hun* stuck in the chimney related to the level of the Triple Warmer at the Lesser Omentum. I assume because that is where the holographic Spirit *Hun* reside, although I suspect that the *hun* may be able to be "stuck" in a number of tissues along the energy meridian, or channel divergencies, anywhere within the *Fire* element, and depending on the location, this could lead to specific manifestations of psychosomatic symptoms.

This is where the Observer's listening skills in clinic will help to decipher the story of what the body is holding, and the origin of the symptom or disfunction.

Regardless of whether one resonates with the *hun* being a flock of bird messengers, or the unlimited sparks of bonfire flames, either archetype may get stuck in the chimney.

Imagine a flock of Swifts nested in a chimney tower, unable to get out due to a blockage of some kind of energy... You may see a slow decline in vitality, and confusion as to where the access to the passions of life has gone... You may see a frantic fluster of the flock agitated, irritated, and angry, unable to fulfill their purpose of connecting to the energy of the world outside the immediate nest. This is the kind of confused agitation that results from an inability to know the reason for being so still, or why they are not even able to see the light of day... It is almost like a Sympathetic kind of depression.

Now imagine a different scenario: the sparkling flames of a fire burning in a fireplace...only the chimney seems to be a little clogged, when all of the sudden some energy comes into the chimney space:

...a burst of flames from the fire, clearing out some organic material that had been hidden in the flue;

...or some resin from the burn that was particularly sticky, causing creosote to collect in the chimney stack until the air flow is reduced to a whisper;

...or perhaps some aggressive rogue birds suddenly disrupting the airflow with a nest made of all kinds of sharp and hurtful things...

I commonly see physical and emotional symptoms of *hun* stuck in the chimney manifest as:

- pain or tension in the hypochondriac area, often confused as "Gallbladder pain;"
- nausea;
- Gastroesophageal sphincter disfunction;
- poor digestion of proteins and fats;
- anxiety;
- lack of self love and self care;
- loss of "intuition;"
- chronic fatigue, or sense of feeling sedentary;
- restlessness;
- depression; and
- loss of a sense of purpose, or the stagnant feeling that you are unable to fulfill your destiny, without a knowing of why.

Physical pain and disfunction attributed to the organs of the *Wood* element may sometimes be caused by physical or energetic restrictions within the *Fire* element, often the Lesser Omentum, especially in the case of emotional stress or trauma.

The Lesser Omentum is the connective tissue that contains the Hepatoduodenal ligament. Restrictions and tension in this area can cause a backup of fluids in the Biliary tree.

Physical and energetic release of the Lesser Omentum often helps free this stagnation, which in turn helps restore the lifting and supportive, energetic flow between the *Fire* element and the *Wood* element. Release of restriction in this area speaks to the *Hun* directly.

Digestive disfunction may also be caused by physical restriction in this area. Restriction here may inhibit proper neural relay and regulation of the Autonomic functions associated with digestion. Also possible is the allowance for emotional holding patterns to develop in this area, creating a stress, further disrupting the balance of the Parasympathetic Dorsal Vagal digestive functions. The potential for this is relative to restriction of the *afferent* neural pathways associated with the Nodose Ganglia, within the Hepatic Hilum of the Hepatoduodenal ligament.

In this case, working directly, gently, with intention, on the tissues of the Lesser Omentum, as well as the Greater Omentum and Small Intestine, may help to release tension and balance pressures within the abdomen, restoring the balance of the internal environment, and allowing for proper transfer of *afferent* neural information.

The Resilience of *hun*

In order for the *hun* to recover their natural state, a state of being a benevolent Observer and witness to the Worlds outside of themselves, the restoration of their comings and goings must be accomplished through a release and integration. For the reincorporation of their purpose of being the bearer of feelings of gratitude and freedom, the *hun* must be well informed, supported, and lifted by the aspects of *shen*, affiliated with the Earth element.

As the function of the *hun* is restored, and a sense of gratitude, support, and safety come back into one's experience, a person may notice:

- a renewed sense of self;
- less negative feelings toward their life situation, and less self judgement;
- the ability to make decisions from a place of love and support, leading to less impulsivity;
- the ability to take responsibility for one's actions;
- the ability to empathize;
- a renewed sense of creativity and passion;
- increased ability to pursue passions and work toward goals;
- a feeling of greater ease;
- the ability to see and feel "your truth;"
- a sense of alignment with purpose;
- a renewed sense of integrity in actions toward others; and
- the ability to truly enjoy and appreciate social connections.

Ideally, the *Earth* element needs to be a welcoming, stable, safe, and supportive presence, for the *hun* to rest easy, in a knowing of the Self, that fosters a healthy Ego. Self care, and Self appreciation, are essential nourishment for the *Soul* and spirit of the *Fire* element.

The voices of the *hun* bring the light of the heavens to the human *Soul*, so that the *zhi* may have support and guidance to manifest Divine Will on the Earth plane. The *hun* are supported and lifted by the *shen* of the *Earth* in this process of negentropic flow of *qì* through the *Tan Cycle*, just as the ground provides the substrate for the roaring of a fire.

The emergence of *empathy* and *benevolence* is a result of the resilience of the Phoenix emerging from the lessons learned within the flames of the fire, marking a right of passage, a leveling up, and healing of the *hun;* a *hun* that is ready to receive.

If we are not provided with stability from the *Earth,* and our primary emotional nourishment early on in life, then we must learn it… often repeating cycles of mentally and emotionally challenging, or even abusive relationships, in order to build contrast and find our way back to our true nature; back to loving and supporting our *Self*…to knowing and *feeling* our true, Divine worth.

Moreover, if the *Fire* element does not receive enough safety and support from the *Earth* element, there is no structure for the *Shen* to nest within its home in the Heart…

When the *hun* are in harmony with the *Shen*, secure within the nest of the Heart, we are able to return to our original nature, the *Te,* as it is known in Taoist tradition. Here the virtues of benevolence and intuition are guided by a pure light of awareness, a *B*eing from the realms of our highest integrity.

The chakra that is associated with the *hun* spirit is the High Heart chakra, corresponding to the Cardiac plexus. When in balance and aligned, this energy center allows us to feel and radiate Divine love and connection to a greater, benevolent, presence that is supportive and nurturing, filled with unconditional love and appreciation for All that is.

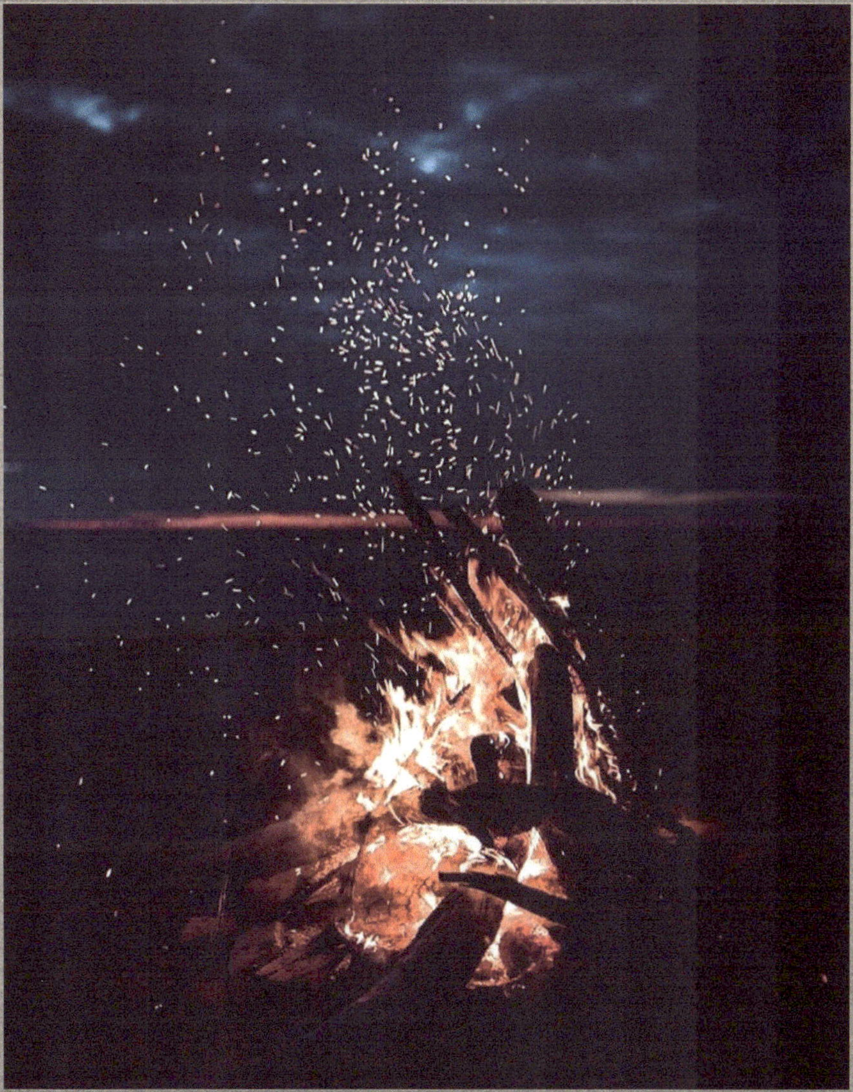

The *Earth* element provides the stable foundation and unconditional support for the *Fire* element to preform alchemical magic. The energy of the *Fire,* the light of transformation, requires a solid base to rest. The *Earth* is consistent, patient, and present; its presence empowers the path of what the *Navajo, the Dine'* people of the North American Southwest, refer to as the "Beauty Way."

To *Walk in Beauty, Ho'zho' Naasha,* means to be at one with,
connected to, and part of, the world around you.
In peace, balance, harmony, and beauty.

When in harmony, mother *Earth* element provides the essential patience and unconditional love, ever present, as boundless joy arises. This is the reason the Spirit of the *Shen* are able to make their home within the Heart.

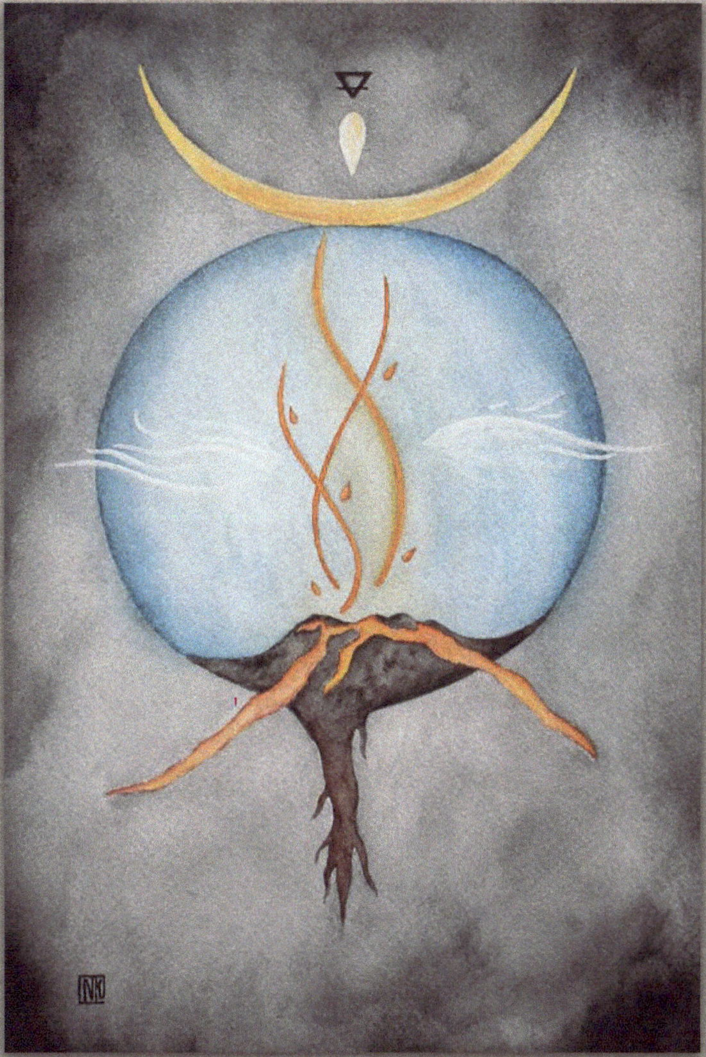

"As Above, So Below," Watercolor © 2021 Nicole Rachelle Keane, Gratitude Healing Arts, LLC

"As above, so below. As within, so without. As the Universe, so the Soul."

– Hermes Trismegistus, 'The Emerald Tablet'

THE CHARACTER FOR *SHEN*

神

"The character *shen* is composed of two elements. On the left, heaven is pictured above the portents of the moon, stars, and sun…On the right are two hands…extending a rope, giving the idea of expansion or extension. Taken as a whole, this character gives the sense of heaven extending its will toward earth and the consciousness of humankind. Humans, in turn, extend their own *shen* toward their *jing* in the act of self-discovery. As the *yang* aspect of the heart spirit, *shen* empowers the creative and expansive nature of heaven within each individual "

- Lonny Jarrett, 'Nourishing Destiny'

Attributes of the Earth Element

Spirit Affiliation - *shen*

Organan officials: Spleen *yin,* Stomach *yang*

"The *Shen* are *yang*. They are polarized toward heaven and their natural tendency is anti-gravitational and negentropic." *(Dachar)* The *shen* are a spirit affiliation that, like the *hun*, is thought of as a flock of birds. They are affiliated with the *Earth* element, but the holographic Spirit *Shen* nest above the Earth, within the *Heart*. The Spirit of *Shen* is able to nest with support from the *shen* of the *Earth* element, and a well regulated Autonomic Nervous System (ANS).

The character for *shen* perfectly illustrates the connection between the Divine illumination of the Cosmos, and life on Earth, reaching toward this glow, reflecting the brilliance of the Divine by manifestation, through inspired action and appreciation of the Self for simply *Be*ing.

Moreover, the character for the *Earth* element is contained within the character for *shen;* the Stomach, the *yang* organ of the *Earth* element, has both expanding and extending qualities, as it takes in nutrients from the outside world, and reaches up, like a rope, past the Heart, toward the Heavens, through the continuous tissue of the Esophagus. The Gastroesophageal sphincter could be seen as the hands that are holding this rope; if the hands are unable to grasp the rope with a solid connection, due to stress or trauma in the human life, this grip weakens and symptoms of reflux or other pathology may ensue, depending on the quality of the disfunction.

The Vagus nerve follows the contour of the Esophagus down through the Diaphragm. This area is of particular importance to the Polyvagal system, as related to the *Five Elements*, because of the location of the Gallbladder Divergent channel, and the overlapping energies of the spirits of *Wood, Fire,* and *Earth.*

"During our lives, the *Shen* are said to reside in emptiness at the center of the heart. From a Chinese medical perspective, the heart is not only a physical organ but also the emperor/empress, the 'supreme sovereign' of the body and mind. The heart, as sovereign, is responsible for the circulation of the blood and the overall state of the emotions as well as the well being of the *shen." (Dachar)*

As the emptiness of the Heart fills with the stresses and traumas of life, the Spirit *Shen* are forced out of their nest, down toward the Earth, and into hiding places near the *yin* Spleen and the *yang* Stomach. I have found in my clinical practice that the *Shen* often hide behind the Stomach, up toward the Spleen, being comforted by the *yin,* mothering, aspects of the Spleen, and drawn in by the polarity of the Feminine *yin* energy.

All of the emotions and disappointments of life may contribute to this abandonment of the nest within the Heart. As the Stomach is the organ that represents the Self in the world around us, if we are in a state of Self-abandonment, due to trauma and post traumatic stress, then the *Earth* element, is not able to lift and support the *Fire* element; the *Shen* may become displaced from the nest as the Heart fills with emotion, unable to integrate, or let go of, the burdens that are collecting within. Our resilience diminishes, and the health of our body and mind suffer greatly.

Early in life, within the first two cycles of growth and renewal, the energetic system of the body is very easily influenced by the qualities of the surrounding environment. The first cycle of growth is from approximately two months prior to the predicted birth date, to approximately seven to eight years of age; the second cycle being from age seven to approximately 14-16 years of age.

This time frame is when our closest relationships to the Other are in the form of the bonds that we have with our primary caregivers, usually the Mother, Father, and siblings; although these energies may take whatever form is relative in the life of the individual, as the nature of family is extremely variable. Family trauma can take on many dimensions, and is spectral in nature.

The way trauma is processed and manifests within an individual is wildly variable, depending greatly on innate physiological or genetic factors, as well as the way environmental stimuli and stress have been collected within the nervous system over time.

Some examples of relationship dynamics that may negatively affect the developing *shen* and the stability of the *Earth* element include:

- premature birth and isolation in the NICU;
- an infant who is deprived of adequate attachment and bonding with a primary caregiver;
- one or both primary caregiver(s) experiencing symptoms of depression that prevent connection and bonding;
- one or both of the primary caregiver(s) being active substance abusers;
- some instances of death of a parent or sibling;
- some instances of traumatic divorce between primary caregivers;
- neglect;
- verbal emotional abuse;
- physical abuse;
- sexual abuse; and
- communication from primary caregivers that is on the Narcissistic spectrum of manipulative behaviors.

The foundations of a strong *Earth* element are essential for our emotional *resilience* in times of stress, providing stability for the *Wood* element and our physical nervous system, through the mediator of the *Fire* element. This triad supports healthy Ventral Vagal ANS regulation.

This is explained through the connection of the *Wood, Fire,* and *Earth* elements to the *afferent* pathway of the Dorsal Vagus. This *Way* begins with the Nodose Ganglia, located in the Hepatic Hilum and area of the Pancreas. The Dorsal Vagal information pathway then reaches up to the Vagal nuclei in the Brainstem. The *afferent* information goes even farther on, to places in the Brain such as the higher order neural connections of the Limbic System and Cortex. The circuit then loops back into the Vagal nuclei of the Brainstem, affecting *efferent* regulation and control of the Autonomic functions of the body.

Of the avian spirits, I feel the *shen* to be less numerous and less ephemeral than the *hun* of the *Fire* element, that are always coming and going. In fact for the body and mind to be healthy and balanced, the *shen,* must stay fairly close to home. As the *hun* have both aviary qualities, as well as those of the flames of a fire, the avian spirit affiliation of *shen,* is also a luminary that has the qualities of a star: having a light that is constant and renewable under the right conditions, with the internal combustion power that radiates directly from Source energy, perpetually renewing and reaffirming itself when in balance.

When the Heart is filled with trauma, the light of the Spirit *Shen* becomes erratic. Instead of having a quality of constant brilliance, it begins to flicker; it grows dark. It is very rare for the *Shen* to actually leave the body altogether while there is still life within; this would cause the Heart to plunge into darkness. Rather they prefer to hide, usually behind the Stomach, near the Spleen, as described.

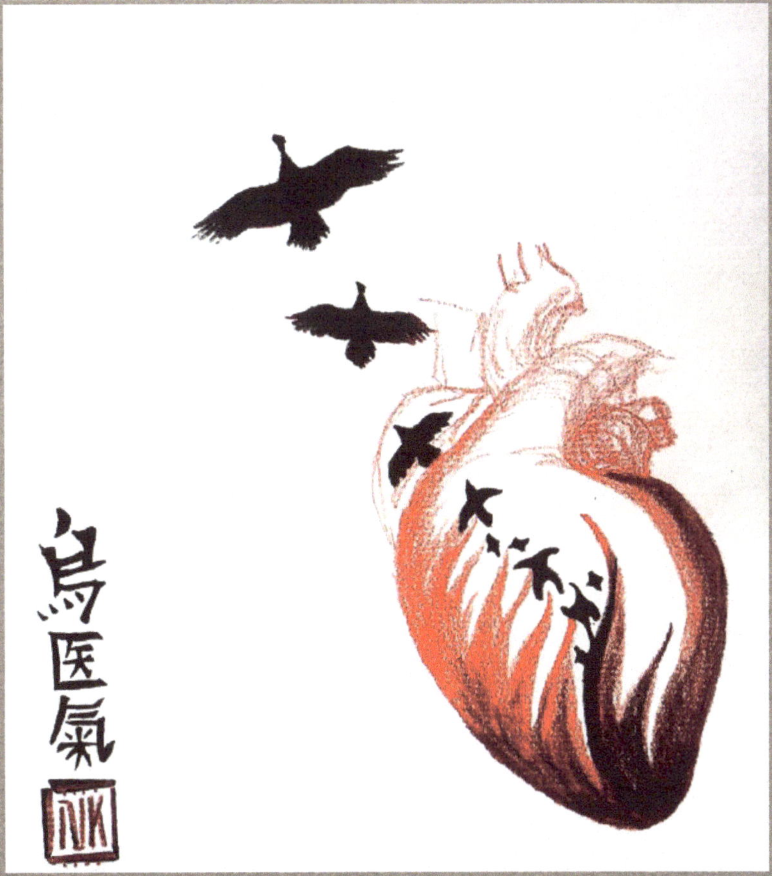

SHEN CLEANING THEIR NEST: THE HEART OF DARKNESS

I channeled this image, drawing it during the tumultuous ending of a relationship which I experienced as abusive. What had started as a warm, gentle relationship evolved into a place of darkness. As that presence gradually started to flood into me, I had an image come into my mind's eye. I saw a small flock of black birds break free from a Heart. I recognize that this image was that of my Shen, and that one day in the future, my Heart would be clear of the darkness that had built up within it during that time.

I started drawing that night and this was the image that ended up on my page; a foreshadowing of the work to be done.

Theoretically, the *Shen* could hide elsewhere within the *Earth* element, including the areas of the Esophagus, Pancreas, and Pylorus. I suppose the more difficult the trauma is to process, the more obscure a place they could be hiding... If the *shen* of the *Earth* element were to become completely depleted and void of any ability to support, causing the Spirit *Shen* to altogether leave the body, this would be a cause of significant psychological pathology, perhaps even sociopathy or psychopathy.

Instability within the *shen of the Earth* element may manifest in symptoms such as:

- anxiety that feels like the rug has been pulled out from under you;
- flares of feeling startled easily;
- sleepless nights due to a pervasive sense of Grief or loss;
- inconsistency, and lack of accountability;
- feelings of victimization;
- poor ability to focus on tasks;
- excessive emphasis on planning, and control orientation toward present situations;
- worry that situations will not turn out as planned;
- oversharing, over giving or inappropriate giving, and talking excessively, especially to people that have not established trust;
- co-dependency typical of "fawn" behaviors;
- being overly focused on fitting into social groups;
- validation seeking behavior; and
- inappropriate emotional responses to interpersonal communication; not necessarily on the spectrum of lack of empathy, but more just an unexpected, or off course, kind of response relative to the context, or gravity of the situation.

The dominant energy of the *Shen* that nest in the Heart is *yang*, or Masculine in nature. When the balanced *yang* aspects of the *Shen* are distorted or compromised by trauma, the polarity can sometimes shift, and the dominant energy of the *Shen* may turn to a distorted *yin*.

This can disturb the polarity that naturally secures the *yang Shen* in their nest within the *yin* Heart. The polarity of the *yang Shen* also anchors their nest toward the *Earth*, and the *yin* energy of the *Yi* within the Spleen, which lies just across the Diaphragm from the Heart. Anatomically, the Heart sits above the Diaphragm, and is oriented toward the Spleen. The presence of distortion, and subsequent reverse of polarity to a dominant *yin*, can repel the *Shen* away from the nest in the Heart, encouraging an act of abandonment, and attracting them to hide behind the Stomach for protection, as the Stomach's dominant energy is *yang*.

With the *Shen* out of harmony with the resonance of the *Earth*, the Soul has a lack of recognition of the Self. This can lead to inconsistencies in behavior, and an inability to embody one's own true nature and integrity. If there is no energetic polarity that supports the individual; one can feel lost in the ethers, blown by the Wind.

In fact, Self-abandonment is a dominant factor for how trauma manifest in the body, and one must have a sure sense of Self to be truly resilient. However, one must have the ability to co-regulate first, before the ability to Self-regulate comes, as we must be able to see into the mirror of the Other, to truly know the Self.

In this mirror, there may be good or bad visions, but it is this contrast, and the awareness it brings, that helps grow the light of the *Shen*, and connect us with our true nature.

Without the stability and assurance, that is offered by a healthy, stable, and unconditional mirror of an Other, we may become detached from our inner knowing and intuition. We may even identify with a false sense of Self and a false intuition.

This becomes apparent in cases of post traumatic stress where an individual identifies with the stressor, and feels more "safe" in the presence of that stress, abuse, chaos, or instability.

This can lead to patterns of toxic interpersonal relationships and difficult challenges in life, as we are forced by the mirror of the Other, to reaffirm our identity, again and again, unable to escape the toxic reflection. These patterns will repeat consistently over a lifetime, until we are awakened by enough Ego death and karmic lessons to draw appropriate boundaries around our domain. The true nature of our Self as the central Emperor or Empress must be rediscovered, and the Divine light of a balanced *Shen* will nest within the Heart once again.

Incredible loss and deep Grief can flow into the *Earth* element from the Lungs of the *Metal/Air* element. This happens when the *Water* element is too week to lift and support the *Metal* element through its virtue of integration. The normally lifting and supporting attributes of the *Metal* element: to process and let go of grief, break down, allowing Grief to permeate through the boundary of the Diaphragm, into the Spleen.

The Spleen is responsible for storing blood and iron for the body, and is one of the prime lymphatic and immune regulators. When burdened from a weak *Metal* element, it becomes heavy with a type of Grief that is encompassing of a deep longing for a life out of reach. The Portuguese have a word for this called "Saudad;" the Grief of yearning for a future never to *Be*.

I have seen in my own life, and in clinical practice, that this may result in a deep restlessness and hopelessness on a primal level. The loss of a significant partnership; or the death or dramatic removal of one's child, or close sibling, due to loss of life, or addiction; results in a death that takes the life of the person still living, still grieving.

This is a very significant Soul level disturbance, and should be treated as such, with reference to the treatment philosophy of the lifting and supporting energy flow of the *Tan Cycle*, as well as respectful use of the *Yu Angles*. This particular set of symptoms being manifest through the *Earth* element, would suggest treatment in an indirect *Way* through the *Wood* and *Water* elements, or more directly through attention to the organs and channels of the *Metal/Air* element.

The *Earth* element lifts and supports the *Fire* element, and extends that energy toward the *Wood* element, empowering each element in the counterclockwise, negentropic energy flow of the *Tan Cycle*.

With regard to anatomical and physiological reference, the Stomach of the *Earth* element, lifts the Greater Omentum of the Triple Warmer of the *Fire* element; and is also lifting and supporting of the first part of the Small Intestine, the Duodenum, which is attached to the Pylorus of the Stomach, and nests together with the Pancreas.

Moreover, with regard to the *Polyvagal Theory*, the Dorsal Vagus follows the Esophagus through the Diaphragm to the Stomach, where it branches out to provide Parasympathetic innervation to the viscera of the abdomen. The Dorsal Vagus needs to be in a healthy, non reactive state, in order to provide a consistency for the light of the *shen* to illuminate the Spirit *Shen*. This harmonic facilitates proper Parasympathetic Ventral Vagal functioning and ANS regulation.

We can see, through these affiliations, how emotional disruption of the *shen* of the *Earth* element, may harm the digestive fire of the Stomach and Pancreas, leading to the inability to properly digest proteins, carbohydrates, and fats; a function related to the digestive enzymes and physiology of the *Earth* element and associated energy channels; this includes lingual enzymes, Stomach acid, as well as Pancreatic enzymes.

This weakness of the *Earth* element sets the stage for inadequate assimilation of nutrients by the Small Intestines of the *Fire* element.

Proteins *are* the foundation of life; together with mineral elements and water, these are the aspects that allow human life to function and flourish. Through cellular structures, ionic charges, and neurotransmitters, we are a quantum reality that is dependent on *Earth*.

The Resilience of *shen*

When the *Shen* are hiding, they are very easy to release into the light of awareness. They do not tend to get stuck in places, like the *Hun,* for they long for the nest of the Heart. Once assured that they are well supported by a healthy sense of Self, they will swiftly take up a mission of re-establishing their nest within the Heart. This is often dependent on energetic and physical liberation of the restrictions within the pathways of the *Earth* element.

The Observer must listen to the tissues of the body to assess and release any physical or energetic restrictions that are preventing the flightpath of the *Shen* toward their home. Examples of techniques associated with this process are given within the *Elemental Manual Meridian Techniques (EMMT)* curriculum that is an accompaniment to this manual.

When the nervous system is in a well regulated and balanced state, we are said to be in Parasympathetic Ventral Vagal regulation, meaning that our emotions are under control, and our ANS is able to function optimally, optimizing our bodily processes and rhythms… We are *resilient,* and we are able to observe, process, and respond, to stress in an appropriate *Way*.

As Pema Chodron says, "You are the sky. Everything else - it's just the weather."

When the nervous system has developed with a lack of support, neglectful treatment, or abuse of any kind, it is much, much harder to be the Sky and watch the clouds go by… when we do not have a solid *Earth* for a reference point, this is a very disorienting experience.

The spirit affiliation of *shen,* as well as the *Shen* Spirit, are inherently very industrious and resilient. Co-regulation with another human being, through a gentle reassuring voice, the soft touch of sincere eye contact, and the healing harmony of laughter, can provide a rhythm for regulation.

A hug and human contact are also very valuable currency.

All of these healing initiators help release Oxytocin, one of the neuroendocrine hormones referenced within the *Polyvagal Theory* as a key regulator of the ANS. It is what allows the human nervous system to experience immobilization *without* Fear.

The *yang* organ of the *Earth* element, the Stomach, lifts and supports the energetic functions of the *yin* Heart, as the primary Stomach meridian crosses the face and interacts with the muscles of facial expression, anchoring our capacity for Social Engagement with others.

This is the basis for the "Face-Heart Connection," referenced in the *Polyvagal Theory,* as a contributing factor to co-regulation and feelings of safety within the presence of another. Our capacity for Social Engagement is a main component in the process of immobilization *without* Fear, which is essential in the function of a healthy, balanced Parasympathetic Vagal system.

Co-regulation with another person, and the Face-Heart connection, is the cornerstone of the Social Engagement System. However, we are not always able to co-regulate. Sometimes the Dorsal Vagal complex is dominant, and we need to do something to calm our Selves so we may return to Social Engagement and Ventral Vagal Regulation.

One technique that can be done to facilitate reconnection with the sense of Self, is to put one hand (whichever is most comfortable) at the area of the Solar Plexus. This chakra is associated with the *Earth* element, and the Celiac and Superior Mesenteric Plexus. The other hand may rest on the area near the lower *dantian*, or the Inferior Mesenteric plexus, that is correlative to the *Metal* element.

Before I begin this technique, I imagine the spiraling Milky Way, our supportive Mother Galaxy; I envision the contraction and expansion cycles of the Universe, and the spiraling, outstretching, nature of that rhythm. "As within, so without, as the Universe, so the Soul…"

Settle yourself in your seat, or with a comfortable standing posture, and gently sink into the rhythm of your breath. You may feel your hands slightly spiral inward. Ease into this collection of your energy, as you follow the contraction of the Universe of energy within you.

Once you have gotten to the end of that contraction cycle, you may feel your body release, and your center start to expand. Follow this movement of energy all the *Way*. Repeat this cycle, with a natural rhythm that feels easy to you. Tune into the breath as you slowly breathe out; allow yourself the patience to complete these cycles in your own time.

As the *shen* of the *Earth* element heals from the trauma of an abusive childhood, or emotional turmoil experienced later in life, the Soul begins to feel safe, back within the Self… an alignment takes place, and resilience approaches ease.

Disturbed *Shen*, more than any of the other Spirits, can lead to perpetual cycles of trauma, and the depolarization of the Masculine and Feminine energies within the body. The *yin* and the *yang* become distorted, and manifest outwardly like the visions within fractured pieces of a glass mirror. As the *Shen* heal, through the support of the spirit affiliation of *shen* and the *Earth* element, so too does the Masculine and Feminine nature. A re-polarization occurs, and balance can be found within the Self. Gradually, the Self comes back home, to ground with the *Earth*, having a greater awareness that is gained from a new, more cohesive joinery within the fault lines of our personality.

"The wound is the place where the light enters you." - Rumi

With the *shen* of the *Earth* element restored, now able to again reflect the light of the *Shen* in the Heart; with this quality of fullness, there may now be a renewed sense of creativity and expression. Where there was previously Distorted Masculine energy, dominating from a necessity for survival; there may now be a balancing of equals, and a rise of the Divine Feminine energy, onto this balance.

One may find that new people enter their life, or that they are able to have deeper connections with the relationships that are currently in their sphere. This is a way that we are able to more completely identify with our "Soul Tribe," as we come into a better understanding of our Self, and are able to radiate that energy outward. We are less distracted by the people and situations that do not resonate with us...we are more focused and discerning, and we may also *receive* guidance to follow our Soul's mission in this life. We have the strength to follow Divine guidance, with unconditional love for the Self, the Journey, and the Other; we follow the *Way*...

When the *shen* is truly balanced, and able to move between *yin* and *yang* energies, there is a soft, quiet, and humble contentment; a shining of beauty that surrounds every powerful step toward the future that will *Be*.

In beauty I walk

With beauty before me I walk
With beauty behind me I walk
With beauty above me I walk
With beauty around me I walk
It has become beauty again

Hózhóogo naasháa doo Shitsijí' hózhóogo naasháa doo Shikéédéé
hózhóogo naasháa doo Shideigi hózhóogo naasháa doo T'áá altso
shinaagóó hózhóogo naasháa doo Hózhó náhásdlíí' Hózhó náhásdlíí'
Hózhó náhásdlíí' Hózhó náhásdlíí'

Today I will walk out, today everything negative will leave me.
I will be as I was before, I will have a cool breeze over my body.
I will have a light body, I will be happy forever, nothing will hinder me.
I walk with beauty before me. I walk with beauty behind me.
I walk with beauty below me. I walk with beauty above me.
I walk with beauty around me. My words will be beautiful.
In beauty all day long may I walk.
Through the returning seasons, may I walk.
On the trail marked with pollen may I walk.
With dew about my feet, may I walk.
With beauty before me may I walk.
With beauty behind me may I walk.
With beauty below me may I walk.
With beauty above me may I walk.
With beauty all around me may I walk.
In old age wandering on a trail of beauty, lively, may I walk.
In old age wandering on a trail of beauty, living again, may I walk.
My words will be beautiful…

From **Walk In Beauty: Prayer From The Navajo (Dine') People**

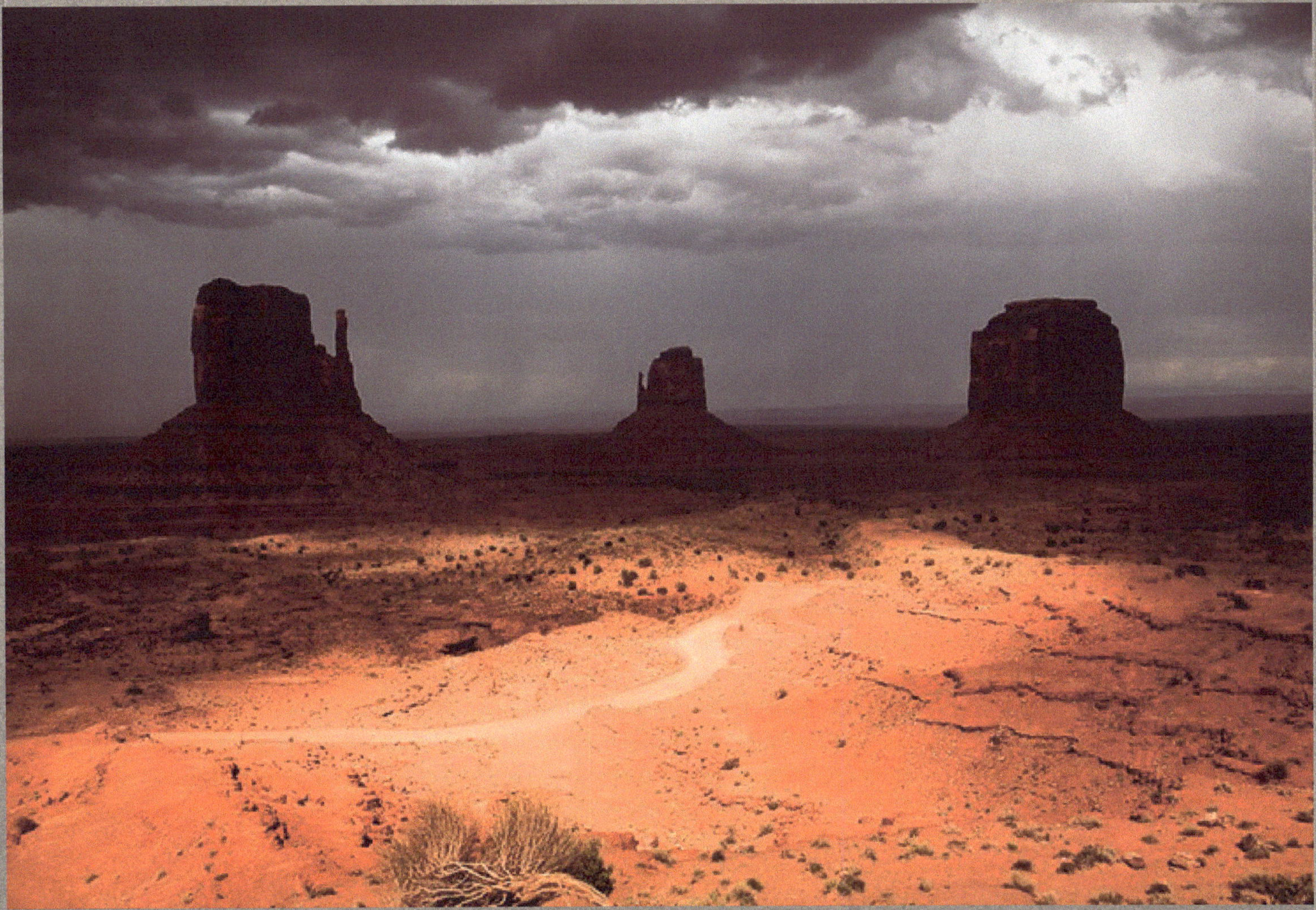

© Peter Zamorowski

The *Metal* element has also been known in various healing traditions as the *Air* element. This chapter will weave together the characteristics of both *Metal* and *Air,* as the quantum nature of anything can be both particle and wave, depending on the Observer. The energy of this element is inextricably linked to the energy of *Earth.* The element of *Metal* lifts and supports *Earth,* as the mantle, and core, of this planet are made of metal.

Metal nourishes the *Earth,* and is found in crystalline form throughout its substrate. *Metal* carries the energy of focused intention, planning, and reciprocity; equal give and take, releasing and receiving.

Together *Metal* and *Earth* form a foundation for the *Fire* of transformation, and the warmth and light of the *Shen,* that is fanned and dispersed through the potentials within *Air.*

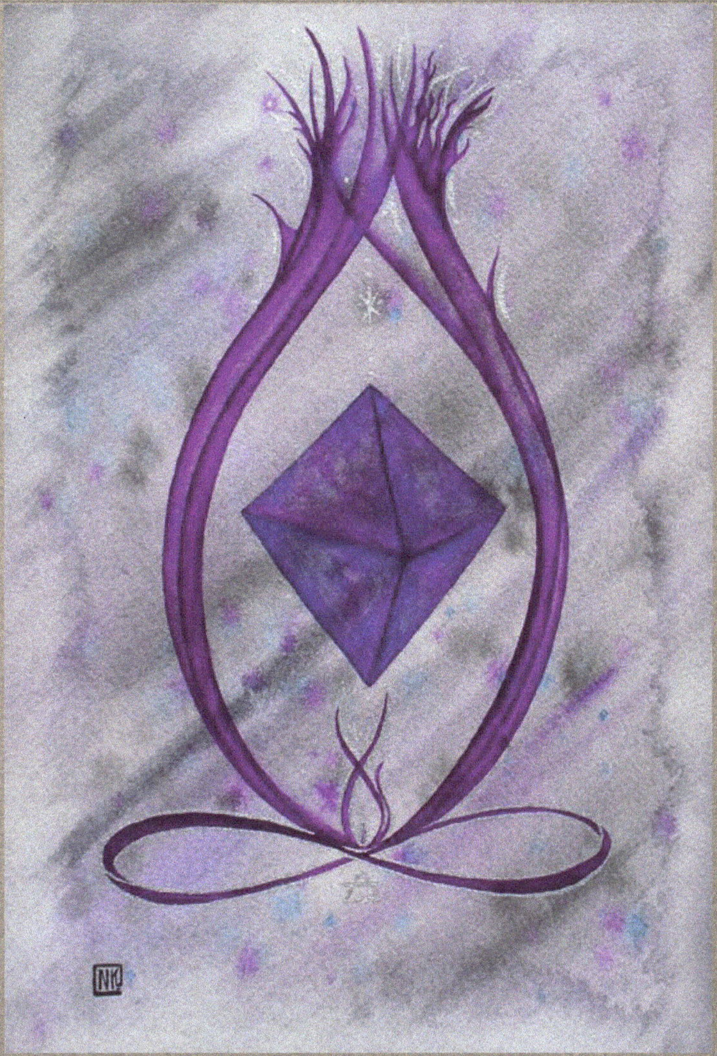

"The Violet Breath," Watercolor © 2021 Nicole Rachelle Keane, Gratitude Healing Arts, LLC

"One of the most ancient words for spirit is the Hebrew word *Ruah;* this is also the word for air or wind. Ruah also denotes pathos, passion, and emotion - a state of the soul. The word suggests that God was like breath and wind because of the incredible passion and pathos of divinity. This ancient recognition links the wild creativity of the Spirit with the breath of the soul in the human person...The world of thought resides in the air... Our greatest thoughts come to us from the generosity of the air. It is here that the idea of inspiration is rooted - you inspire or breath in the thoughts concealed in the air element. You can prepare, making yourself ready to be inspired, yet it is spontaneous and unpredictable... Inspiration is always a surprising visitor. "

– John O'Donoghue, 'Anam Cara: A Book of Celtic Wisdom'

THE CHARACTER FOR *YI*

意

"The character *yi* shows us the picture of the open bowl of the heart. Above it is the radical indicating an uttered sound, poetry or a musical note. Sound is vibration. Like the Wind, sound creates movement through the air, a breeze. Like the wind, it is a messenger between realms. Sound, in the form of prayers, chanting and poetry, carries our hopes and desires into the world and up to the heavens"

-Lori Eve Dachar, 'Five Spirits'

Attributes of the Metal or Air Element

Spirit Affiliation - *yi*

Organ officials: Lung *yin,* Large Intestine *yang*

The *Metal or Air* element is the first element that we approach as we trace backward through the *Tan Cycle,* traveling below the horizon to enter the Underworld of the *Five Elements. Metal* carries a density of memories, and is tasked with recollecting, assessing, and integrating the information received from living.

The *yin* organ of the Lung carries out the task of taking in the environment through the breath. Further refinement of the environment experienced: the purpose, assimilation, and letting go of what no longer serves us, happens through the *yang* organ of the *Metal* element, the Large Intestine, but also through the *yang* qualities of the Lung. With the voice and breath, the Lungs have a function of letting go, as the out breath releases internal environmental toxins collected within the blood; likewise, our voice on the wind has the potential to provide a cleansing of emotional toxins that have collected within the Heart and Mind, a release and renewal created by speaking One's truth.

Both the characters for *zhi* (*Wood* element) and *yi* (*Metal/Air* element) contain the radical for Heart. I interpret this to relate to the properties of the spirit of *Metal* to support and lift the Spirit of *Yi,* that resides within the Spleen of the *Earth* element. The Spirit *Yi* provides essential nourishment and polarity for the *Shen* of the Heart to thrive. With the Heart being in a position of strength, it is available for a healthy manifestation of the *zhi*, or Divine Will of the *Wood* element; allowing for the view of a supportive and balanced path to healing from trauma.

The sound of *yi* is like the slow resonant harmonic of a crystal singing bowl. It has a sound that surrounds. It is both above and below, and as such, the *yi* are able to assist with a rhythm of regulation for the Autonomic Nervous System (ANS). This background of energetic support lifts the *Fire* and *Wood* elements, allowing for Ventral Vagal regulation of the body and the emotions.

Physiologically the *yi* and *zhi* are both intricately related to the Ventral and Dorsal Vagal pathways; which, when free of restriction, are responsible for proper ANS regulation of the Heart. The resilience of the Vagus nerve, and relative health of the Parasympathetic Ventral Vagal regulatory system, also known as "Vagal tone," is directly correlative to Respiratory Sinus Arrhythmia (RSA) and Heart Rate Variability (HRV). These metrics refer to the variation in amplitude of the Heart rate, in relation to the breath of the Lungs.

This quantifiable variable is considered to be a reliable indicator of physiological levels of resilience within the ANS, and can reliably predict potentials for emotional regulation, histological healing, inflammation, and immune response.

"The *yi* empowers the integration into self of only that which corresponds to the template provided by our inherited constitution" (*Jarrett, Nourishing Destiny).* The state of the *yi* is an indicator of our innate resilience, and is a product of our genetics, as well as the environment that we are born into. This is the essence of our inherited and our acquired constitutions.

The prenatal environment, as well as the support and/or toxicity that we experience as part of our early years through our relationship to our primary caregivers, has a large influence on how our nervous system develops; this happens beyond our conscious cognition, processed and integrated within the depths of our being.

The holographic Spirit of *Yi* takes up residence in the *yin* organ of the Spleen, within the *Earth* element.

The Pancreas is often paired energetically with the Spleen, much like how the elements of *Air* and *Metal* occupy a corresponding place in *Four* and *Five Element* healing traditions. Energetically they are very similar in ways, for their role in the larger picture of the energetic system they exist within; however, they are also very different in how they fulfill their role, regarding specific elemental correspondences, and physiological function.

In this way, the Spirit of *Yi* within the Spleen, is to the element of *Metal;* as the *Yi* of the Pancreas is to the element of *Air*. The density and purpose of the Spleen: storing Iron and supporting immune functions, fulfills an important energetic role in the fertility of the *Earth* element, linking it to the supportive functions of the *Metal* element.

Moreover, the omnipresent neuroendocrine and exocrine functions of the Pancreas, are essential for renewal, as well as sustaining the growth process and future potentials of the *Earth* element, insofar as *Air (*i.e. atmosphere) is essential to the expansion of terrestrial life.

The *yi* within the *Metal/Air* element provide access to the quantum potential available from the material minerals (the *Self),* and the immaterial essence (the *Soul);* both are an embodiment of the energetic characteristics of *Metal* and *Air*. With the holographic Spirit domicile in the *yin* of the *Earth,* the Spirit *Yi* enrich the human experience within our internal and external Universes.

...And as the element of *Metal* is contained within meteorites, the spirit affiliation of *yi* is also the voice and breath of Universes.

Within the *Tan Cycle,* the element of *Metal/Air* has the function of lifting and supporting the *Earth* element. By anatomical proximity and energetic relation, the Splenic flexure of the *yang* Large Intestine diverges slightly from its descending trajectory to energetically support and lift the Spleen. There is also an intimate relationship between these two organs with regard to immune function.

The quantum communications and "cross talk" between organs has been well established in Western medicine. The fascial network, as well as circulatory and nervous systems, carry neuroendocrine messages between tissues, and the composition of the inner microbiome also produces chemical signals that travel on these pathways. A good diversity of beneficial bacteria and fungi within the digestive tract, specifically the Large Intestine, creates opportunity for resonance, and harmonizes energetically with the immune potentials of the Spleen.

Likewise, when there is an imbalance, or overgrowth, within the microbiome, this results in an energetic disturbance that can create an imbalance within the immune functions of the Spleen, potentially having a ripple effect through the entire internal ecosystem. When the Large Intestines are compromised by parasites, or pathological microbial overgrowth, the flexures may be particularly affected, due to their shape and proximity to the Liver and Spleen.

In cases of inflammation of the Splenic flexure, the Spleen and general immune function will be profoundly affected. The *Metal* element will be unable to support and lift the *Earth* element, due to distortion in the Masculine *yang* energy, leading to a breakdown in functioning support that is essential for the *yin* energy of the *Earth.* Moreover, the systemic imbalance that this causes will also affect the *yin* energy of the Lungs, and may result in symptoms of allergies and asthma.

Herein lies a question of how did this begin? In the case of a parasitic infection, likely it resulted from an interaction with the external environment. However, what were the energetic and physical conditions that weakened the immune system, or restricted the physical body from allowing the organism to move through without harm. What lead to the establishment and proliferation of the pathology?

In the case of a microbial overgrowth, what were the conditions that allowed for that pathogen to flourish and proliferate?... When there is a microbial overgrowth, or type of biofilm within the intestines, the Large Intestine is not able to absorb nutrients to support the greater ecosystem within the body.

In order to provide an environment where a pathogen can flourish, the body must be resonating at that same level. If the opposite was the case, the immune system would be able to manage the assault; infection, proliferation, and pathology would not have the opportunity to occur.

When there are problems with elimination, there is often also an emotional, or energetic component that compromises the stability of the whole, affecting the digestive process.

This is an energetic nexus between the *yi* of the *Metal* element, and the holographic Spirit *Yi* that resides within the Spleen, extending to the digestive functions of the Pancreas.

In order for the *Metal/Air* element to function properly, it must have the lifting and supportive energy of the element of *Water*. At its most basic essence, this refers to simple hydration. Hydration and flow assist the *yang* Large Intestine with its most important function, that of releasing emotional and physical toxins, and letting go.

When the *Metal* element is unable to lift and support the *Earth* through properly oxygenating the blood through the Lungs; and unable to carry out the functions of assimilating nutrients and letting go of what does not serve us; and unable to resist stagnation through proper functioning of the Large Intestine; the organs of the *Earth* element, the Spleen, Pancreas, and Stomach, will suffer.

On a physical level, the Observer could see poor digestion, and elevated blood sugar, due to disruption of the neuroendocrine and exocrine functions of the Pancreas and Stomach. Also, depression and muscle spasms could occur, as amino acid and B-12 levels drop, due to insufficient digestion and assimilation of proteins, vitamins, and nutrients, affecting the nerves and neuroendocrine system.

On an energetic level, the most prominent manifestation of *Metal/Air* unable to support *Earth* would be the spectrum of emotion associated with obsessive thoughts, including worry about an uncertain future. Worry is commonly attributed to the Spleen, but it is an emotional distortion rooted within a deficiency of the planning and structuring energy that is part of the essence of *yi*, the spirit affiliation of the *Metal/Air* element. With a strong *Metal/Air* element, we are able to use patience in realization of potential, we are able to be the Sky, and all the worries will pass like the weather.

A Weak *yi* and the Gravitational Precipitation of Grief
(Processing Complex Grief)

On an energetic level, a weak *yi* facilitates the gravitational precipitation of grief, and a breakdown in the grieving process. The *yin* Lungs are the organ that receives and processes grief. If the *yi* are not strong, this could lead to Lung infections on a physical level, as the energy of this emotion can cause the *Metal/Air* element to become stagnant and still, affecting the immune system…

If the *yang* organ of the *Metal* element, the Large Intestine, is too weak to adequately support the processing of grieving and letting go, or is not given enough space to do so, because of physical or energetic restrictions, then the Grief will try to leave the Lungs anyway that it can.

This entrapment, leading to the gravitational precipitation of grief, can happen due to too much of a Sympathetic Nervous System (SNS) stress response, which is caused by a *Water* element that is overwhelmed and unable to integrate stressful experiences.

When the *Water* element is unable to lift and support the *Metal* element, just as water that is too overwhelmed with heat cannot suspend metal within a solution, the energy within *Metal* naturally precipitates out of the fluid matrix of the body, settling into the more dense structures below.

This breakdown in the support process creates an energetic loop of negative feedback, that is kicked off by a SNS response to the emotional processing of grief. The SNS response is attributed to a *Water* element our of balance, and weakness in the Kidney and Adrenal glands.

This feedback loop will eventually lead to the unprocessed emotion collecting in the Kidneys, resulting in severely weakened *qì*.

When Grief cannot flee the Lungs during healthy emotional processing, with respect for the gravity the situation, it begins to settle out of the tissues, sinking into the subconscious, below the Diaphragm, into Dorsal Vagal territory.... Grief that has the quality of Anger will settle toward the Right side of the body, first entering through the Bare Area of Liver that has a direct connection to the Diaphragm.

When aspects of Grief that have an angry quality affect the density of the Liver, they have an opportunity to once again leave the body through the energetic connections of the ligaments of the Hepatic flexure of the Large Intestine. This depends on the *yang* Large Intestine being strong enough, physically and energetically, to process the emotional load. This ability of the Large Intestine very much depends on the strength of the *Water* element, to lift and support that flow.

Physically, the lower part of the Large Intestine, the Sigmoid Colon and Rectum, are not innervated by the Vagus nerve. Rather, they receive Autonomic innervation from the Sacral plexus, which is very much linked to the Sympathetic stress response, and can suffer very easily from distortion in *yin* and *yang* energies.

If the Grief is not able to be processed through the Large Intestine while it is in the Liver, it may lead to imbalance within the *Wood* element, affecting Parasympathetic Ventral Vagal regulation. Symptoms can include Heart palpitations, as well as other imbalances and pathology attributed to *Wood* element disfunction.

Angry Grief can live in the Liver for a very, very long time. The Liver has great capacity for regeneration and renewal. As the Liver processes angry Grief, one may experience symptoms of weakness, fatigue, pain on the right side, and reduced range of motion in the Right shoulder.

The Liver may even be able to process out the toxin of angry Grief by itself, through the physical release of bile; however, being in this type of Masculine, *yang,* energy is particularly taxing for the dominant *yin* energy of the Liver. Moreover, bile infused with Grief is particularly toxic for the Gallbladder to receive and hold. The *yin,* or receptive, energy of the Gallbladder may not be strong enough to receive and process this density, as the Gallbladder is an organ that is naturally *yang*. This may cause the energetic toxin to be dispersed over the Gallbladder Divergent channel, negatively affecting the anatomy and physiology of this pathway, which is of particular importance to Parasympathetic Ventral Vagal regulation.

If angry Grief is not able to leave the body, eventually it will settle, by energy transfer, through the Posterior Coronal ligament of the Liver, into the Right Kidney. Now this is where it gets really deep...because disfunction in the Right Kidney can be caused not only by trauma in this life, but also by intergenerational trauma. In other words, angry Grief that has been passed down epigenetically through generations.

This could happen through emotional and physical abuse patterns that play out within families, from parent to child, as well as energetic transfer from the quantum messages encoded in our DNA. Such transfer could be associated with congenital pathology. Yes, this is absolutely possible, and part of the Universal Law of Conservation of Energy. This is a *Way* genes can get "turned on" and "turned off" for healthy function or pathology. This is our quantum reality.

Now, for the type of Grief that is like the ever present sadness of deep loss... This quality of Grief is sometimes felt as ephemeral, less dense than the qualities of *Metal*, and more like the energy of sinking *Air*; it is like a breath that has been taken from you.

This was talked about with regard to the Spleen, and the emotion of Saudad: the sadness of a future that is unable to *Be*... When the Lungs are not able to process a Grief such as this, the energy will sink, passing near the Heart, through the Diaphragm, and into the Spleen.

Symptoms can include Heart palpitations of a quality similar to heavy drops of water into a deep well, as well as other symptoms of Splenic and Pancreatic disfunction. Importantly, with this specific type of emotional processing, there may be a decrease in the absorption of the vitamin B-12. This occurs through inadequate digestion and assimilation of amino acids that assist in the utilization of B-12, and can lead to a feeling of depression that has the qualities of hopelessness.

Again, here is a juncture where this deep Grief of sadness can leave the body through the Large Intestine, by way of the ligaments of the Splenic flexure of the Large Intestine. If this does not happen, the Pancreas or Stomach may try to process this emotion for the Spleen with the *yang* qualities of their energy. This may lead to pathology of the Pancreas or Stomach, as well as chronic immune pathology, digestive disfunction, and pernicious anemia.

If the Grief of deep sadness is not processed, it will precipitate into the Left Kidney through the energetic pathway within the Splenorenal Ligament. Here it will cause extreme fatigue and diminishment of *qì*. Because the Left Kidney is fascially connected to the arterial blood supply of the reproductive system, fertility and reproductive function may be affected, as well.

If there is mysterious disfunction of the Left Kidney, or potentially a congenital pathology, the cause may be relative to unprocessed Grief that a person has directly experienced in this life, or energy that may have been passed down through generations of unprocessed trauma.

When Grief settles all the way down into the Kidneys, it affects the *po* spirit affiliation of the *Water* element. It becomes embedded into the personality and physical experience. Once gone so far, it is possible that this Grief may not be resolved in this lifetime without energetic intervention, becoming a spoke in the wheel of Karma…

As the body attempts to energetically process complex Grief through moving the energy through the tissues of the body, the *yang* aspect of the *Water* element may be called upon to manage a healthy recovery. By initiating a reversal from Parasympathetic Dorsal Vagal immobilization to a supportive Sympathetic state, the self regulating Parasympathetic Ventral Vagal system is better able to step in and initiate regulated healing.

When the energy that flows along the primary Bladder meridian and Divergent channel is free of physical or energetic restrictions, then the *Water* element, at any time in this process can come "on line" in a supportive way, gently freeing this entropic, decaying, sinking energy of Grief within the physical system.

This is done by activating the gentle warmth of the Heart, through the Bladder Divergent channel, creating a glow within the *Fire* element, and establishing an ease into the supportive functions of *Wood* lifting *Water.* This activates the Parasympathetic Ventral Vagal regulatory system, and can lead to enlightened emotional processing, and the ability to receive the light of the Spirit *Shen,* from their nest within the Heart.

"Grief's role in your healing process is to allow hurt, disappointment, rage, disbelief, and sorrow to move through your body. Trapped emotions create disharmony. They are firmly lodged and sticky. Examine your heartbreaks, the canyons left by emotions that carved you like the Rio Grande. What stories are held in the caverns? What floods have you never allowed to come, for fear they wouldn't stop?...The ghosts of ungrieved pain haunt our inner halls, project onto our loved ones, clog our heart valves, and suck lubrication right out of our joints. Untended, their pressing messages and desperate pleas for flow, slow forward movement."

– Pixie Lighthorse, 'Goldmining the Shadows'

Neuroception, Interoception, and the *yi* and *po* Spirit Affiliations

The *yi* are like a group of mature cultivators, that help to nurture the *Earth* and keep it fertile; they have a perspective gained by their connection to the Underworld and the *Metal* element, as well as the energetic qualities of the omnipresent *Air*. They are seasoned from experience and shaped by the weather of life. They have a knowing beyond our consciousness, and are relative to the concept of *neuroception* in the *Polyvagal Theory*. Moreover, many of the physical and sensory reactions, called "Vasovagal Reflexes," that may occur as a result of *neuroception*, are considered to be symptomatic within the *Metal/Air* element.

The process of perception that happens within our conscious awareness is called Interoception, and is most correspondent with the physical sensing that correlates with the element of *Water*, and the spirit affiliation of *po*.

"Neuroception is the process through which the nervous system evaluates risk without requiring awareness. This automatic process involves brain areas that evaluate cues of safety, danger, and life threat. Once these are detected via neuroception, physiological state automatically shifts to optimize survival. Although we are usually not aware of cues that trigger neuroception, we tend to be aware of the physiological shift (i.e., interoception). Sometimes we experience this as feelings in our gut or heart, or as an intuition that the context is dangerous. Alternatively, this system also triggers physiological states that support trust, social engagement behaviors, and the building of strong relationships. *Neuroception is not always accurate. Faulty neuroception might detect risk when there is no risk, or identify cues of safety when there is risk.*" *(Porges, The Polyvagal Theory)*

Interoception is described in the *Polyvagal Theory* as: "the process describing both conscious feelings and unconscious monitoring of bodily processes by the nervous system. Interoception, similar to other sensory systems, has four components: 1) Sensors located in internal organs to evaluate internal conditions; 2) Sensory pathways conveying information from the organs to the brain; 3) Brain structures to interpret sensory information and to regulate the organ's response to the changing internal conditions; and 4) Motor pathways that communicate information from the brain to the organs, to change the state of the organs. In Polyvagal Theory interoception is the process providing the signal to the brain of changes in physiological state (see Porges, 1993). In contexts in which there are cues of risk or safety, interoception would occur after the process of neuroception. Interoception may result in a conscious awareness of a bodily response. In contrast, neuroception occurs outside conscious awareness" (*Porges, Polyvagal Theory*)

"Interoception reflects the feedback from our viscera to our brain. When we understand interoception, we understand that feedback from different physiological states promotes access to different areas of the brain, and influences decision-making, memory retrieval, and other cognitive processes." *Id.*

The *yi* and the *po* reside in the subterranean space of the *Tan Cycle;* they are familiar with the subconscious. The function of breathing, afforded by the Lungs, is something that happens beyond our consciousness, without requiring awareness; while at the same time breathing is an ever present part of the experience that we are having. In this way, it is like the process of neuroception. It is reflexive.

However, when we are made aware of the action and abilities, the potentials, of the breath, we are able to understand more about our experience, and are consciously able to modify our innate reactions through this liminal space of interacting with the subconscious.

The ability to receive our nervous system's interpretation of our experience of the outside world, to become aware of the innate rhythm in which our body responds to a stimulus, beyond our conscious awareness, is a way that we may attempt to break habitual patterns of trauma in our lives. We may establish an understanding, so that we may avoid self judgement.

If our nervous system has survived significant, chronic trauma, then we may feel more "safe" and comforted within that cycle of trauma, neglect, toxicity, or chaos. This happens because our nervous system does not know a reality beyond this dramatic experience.

Alternatively, when we are presented with a situation of support and loving energy, we may feel very uncomfortable or anxious about that experience... We are aware that something feels "off," and we may become suspicious; we may take paths away from the safety of surrendering into the support offered, and instead choose a self sabotaging path that feels "right" to us, only to be hurt again. We deny ourselves the choice of the path of healing and unconditional acceptance.

Some people experience support and love as very, very disturbing. This is interoception, and an activation of our inner awareness through the Sympathetic stress response.

Within this thought process, it is important to acknowledge that every person's experience of trauma is their own. We must have an awareness that a trauma, as an experience, is held in specific ways within the body, and this is entirely subjective to the individual.

We may not understand why a person feels, or acts, a certain way; in fact, that person may not understand it themselves. This is why it is so very important to approach others with empathy.

"Empathy fuels connection; sympathy drives disconnection." - Dr. Brene' Brown

Theresa Wiseman, a nursing scholar, identified four attributes of empathy:

- Perspective taking - This refers to attempting to come to the same level as the person experiencing the stressful moment; to *Be* with them, in their perspective of their experience.
- Staying out of judgement - This serves as a supportive reminder that each person's experience is their own... and that experience is colored by how previous experiences of stress have influenced their nervous system. This is having an awareness of how the concepts of neuroception and interoception are at work within an individual. It is what is referred to as "holding space."
- Recognizing the emotions of others - This is a call for us to attempt to identify with how a person is feeling by recognizing an experience of our own that may have caused a similar emotion. This requires a great degree of vulnerability, and a willingness to really connect with anOther, and be seen for our true Selves.
- Communicating support and validation - This describes another level of vulnerability, where we are allowing for a genuine connection within the space that has been created, offering true support and validation of the other person's suffering.

The sacred space that can be created by welcoming the presence of true empathy, and supporting the gentle awareness of another person's trauma, can be very healing... and is a continual practice of our ability to connect in a genuine *Way*.

The Resilience of *yi*

The energy of the *Metal/Air* element provides exceptional power for manifestation. It is the solid structure of crystalline forms, and is related to our mineral bones. The essence of both *Metal* and *Air*, are both the structure, as well as the space that fills it, respectively.

In his book *The Web That Has No Weaver*, Ted Kaptchuk, refers to the spirit affiliation of *yi as the "Consciousness of Potentials." He writes, "[yi]* has the task of enabling and supporting new manifestations to come into being. Because the *yi* is insightful, it can understand others, and be generous and extremely aware of the needs of other people and situations. It can see both what can, and what needs to be done."

The *yi* spirit affiliated with the *Metal/Air* element is very industrious, making *Metal/Air* inherently resilient.

While the Spirit *Yi*, at home within the Spleen, has a tendency to stagnate and become slow when in disfunction, it is backed up by the *Metal* element's vibration of shining resiliency, reflecting the beams of the *shen* back onto to the *Earth* element, in support. All that is required to heal a distorted *Yi* is the light of awareness reflecting up from the *yi* of the Large Intestine: this is the Wisdom of letting go. Or as Pema Chodron so clearly puts it, "The Wisdom of No Escape."

This relates to the concept of "Radical Acceptance." When we practice radical acceptance, we are simultaneously activating all aspects of the *yi* spirit affiliated with the element of *Metal/Air*. In fact, we are embodying the essence of both *yin* and *yang* energies by taking in an experience, feeling it, letting it move through us, and letting it go… all at the same time! This is not easy.

It is at once both the end of hope, and the beginning of hope. It is both complex and very simple. It is surrender into the *Tao*. This is an incredibly powerful alchemization practice, and it does take practice.

When you reach the end of hope, you have come to a place of *Wēijī;* this point almost always involves going through the process of grieving to get through to the beginning of a new hope for the future, and a new timeline... This becomes a mental and visceral awareness of your Consciousness of Potentials.

For the act of Radical Acceptance to work, we must really *feel* the thing that has affected us, and *really* Let. It. Go... no dissociation, no rationalization, no dissolusion; if not seen to completion, the emotion and energy of the experience will get stuck in the tissues of the body, along energy pathways that have restriction, and cause disfunction. This energy will stay in a holding pattern, as kinetic energy, waiting to be processed by the body; it is potential energy creating potential patterns of chaos.

Radical Acceptance is a judgement free activity, and it is a practice. Once the process of Radical Acceptance is mastered, it can feel like turning the emotional density of *Metal* into *Air*. It is a kind of Magic.

Along the path of Radical Acceptance, I have found the practice of Tonglen is quite a good stepping stone. Pema Chodron has a small pocket sized book about this process that I love almost as much as my pocket sized book of the *I Ching*. The pages of both of them have nearly turned from particle to wave after all of the years of activity.

The practice of Tonglen goes something like this:

- Find a comfortable position.
- Start broad: Think of something that is expansive and somewhat removed from your personal experience. For instance, wildfires in the Amazon.
- Pick an aspect of suffering that is associated with that issue; such as the loss of life from habitat destruction.
- Now take a moment to imagine that suffering. Breathe it in, through one deep breath.
- As the expansiveness of your inhale and awareness grows, pause; feel that suffering and turmoil; imagine what that heat must feel like; then visualize a bright luminary shining into your chest where that breath is, where all the suffering is; now invite that suffering to be cleansed by that reflective light and welcome it into a place of Love; breath out a resonance of peace and harmony, to all spirit Souls affected by that tragedy.

Once you have done this a few times toward something general, for "the Collective," then you can gradually try to make the subject more personal. Be patient with yourself, and allow the feelings to flow into you, meet them with light and invite them into Love; breathe them out.
Let. Them. Go.

Interestingly, these forms and practices of Radical Acceptance are very similar to the Buddhist lineage of Vajrayiana, also called "the Diamond Vehicle." Of all the Buddhist schools, this is said to be the most challenging, and is rooted in Tantric practices of transformation and alchemy... and this practice happens to have a name synonymous with a crystalline structure...the Diamond, having the character of the *Metal* element.

An exercise that can be done to strengthen the *yi,* and aid in the quest for Radical Acceptance, is to walk or hike briskly, activating the Lungs and the Heart. While in motion, bring the pad of the index finger to the tip of the thumb, in a comfortable mudra position. This will activate the energy flow between the Lung and the Large Intestine meridians of the thumb and index finger, respectively.

Be mindful to breath low, deep into the bottom of the Lungs; this will activate the Diaphragm, and the energy will flow into the Large Intestine from there for processing.

If you find that you are experiencing tingling or numbness in your fingers, this likely means that you are breathing too "high." Try to consciously shift your breath lower. This sensation happens because the Scalene muscles in your neck are working too hard to lift your ribs to allow for expansion of the top of your Lungs; this creates tightening around your Thoracic Inlet.

Sound is also plays an important role in the resilience of *yi,* and offers an opportunity to tonify the Vagus nerve.

Bats are an amazing example of sound vibration attenuating Vagal tone. Bats can live to be 40 years old, much longer than other mammals their size, due to the extremely low levels of inflammation within their bodies. These low levels of inflammation are result of extremely high Vagal tone. The use of echolocation, a form of sonar, for navigation and communication, recruits many of the Craniofacial nerves and Vagal nuclei for processing, developing and toning the Polyvagal system.

This inherently high Vagal tone is precisely why viruses that evolve, and incubate, in bat populations can be so inflammatory within humans. Humans have a much less evolved Polyvagal system. Interestingly, bats are also the only mammal capable of sustained flight through the *Air*.

The Vagus nerve has motor branches that innervate the Vocal cords in the Larynx, as well as areas within the middle ear, and Pharynx. All of these areas have evolved and adapted within Bats, to great degree, specifically for the creation of very high frequency sound, receptivity to sensation, and the precision required for successful use of echolocation.

Singing, listening, and feeling the vibrations of sound can help create resilience, tone the Vagus nerve complex. Ultimately, this leads to higher Vagal tone, increased resilience, and decreased inflammation, especially within the Lungs.

Listening to the song of a Tibetan singing bowl, or the harmonic of a Quartz crystal bowl, can be particularly healing to the *Metal/Air* element, and the *yi*. Sounds in the vocal range of the human voice also sooth the *yi*.

On the other end of the spectrum, low frequency sound, even a very deep human voice, is perceived as a primal threat to survival, and elicits a Sympathetic stress response that negatively affects the *po* spirit affiliated with the *Water* element. Sounds of low droning machinery are a particularly powerful stimulus for the primal Fear and stress reactions that may be neuroceptively triggered, sometimes on a daily basis, without our awareness.

Part of the beauty of the *yi,* and the *Metal/Air* element, lies in the interconnectedness it has with the *Earth* element. When out of balance both the *Earth* element, and the *Metal/Air* element may lead to behaviors on the spectrum of co-dependency.

When in balance, these elements facilitate the formation of interdependent relationships that are the embodiment of the spectrum of true Love... and one of the most lovely aspects of relationships like these is the beauty of reciprocity.

When we are able to have solid, stable, and balanced, *Earth* and *Metal/Air* energies, then we are able to know our inherent value. We are able to appreciate the worth that we have, just for *Being,* and we become versed in how to express our needs and boundaries within relationship, from a place of Grace. We are also able to *receive*.

"Become an alchemist.
Transmute base metal into gold,
suffering into consciousness,
disaster into enlightenment"

- Eckhart Tolle

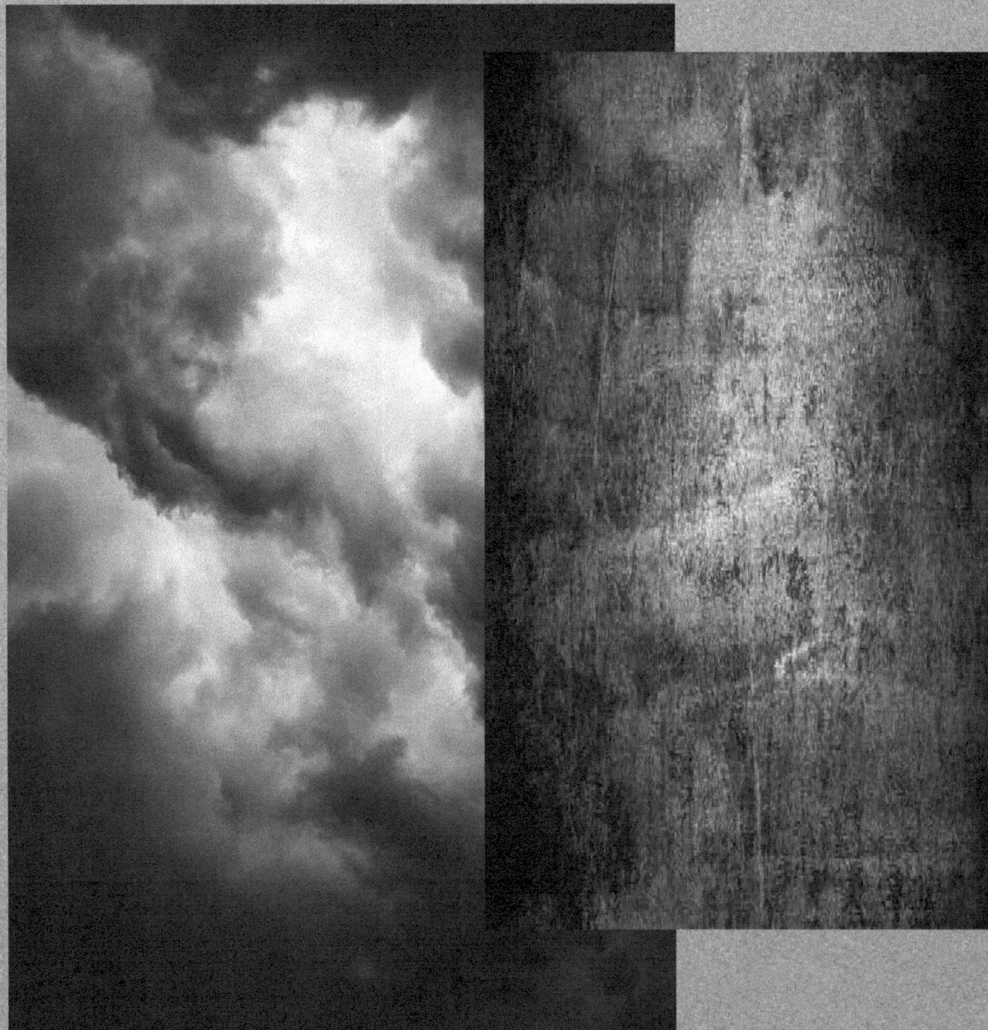

The *Water* element, and the spirit affiliation of *po*, lift and support the *Metal/Air* element. In nature *Metal* dissolves into, and is suspended within, *Water;* likewise, as *Water* transforms into steam, it takes on the qualities of *Air*, intermingling, as the molecules within sublimate into vapor.

Both the *Water* element, and the element of *Metal/Air,* are located below the horizon line of the *Tan Cycle,* within the subterranean space, the subconscious. They have properties that are characteristic of both density and light, depending on the environment. Both *Water* as well as *Metal,* have the ability to reflect, and to change state with ease, given the proper energy and assistance. Both have the potential for great brilliance and great resilience. While *Metal/Air* carries a density that gently guides us into the darkness of the subconscious, the flow of *Water* has the potential to take us out of the caves, and into the light of the Sun.

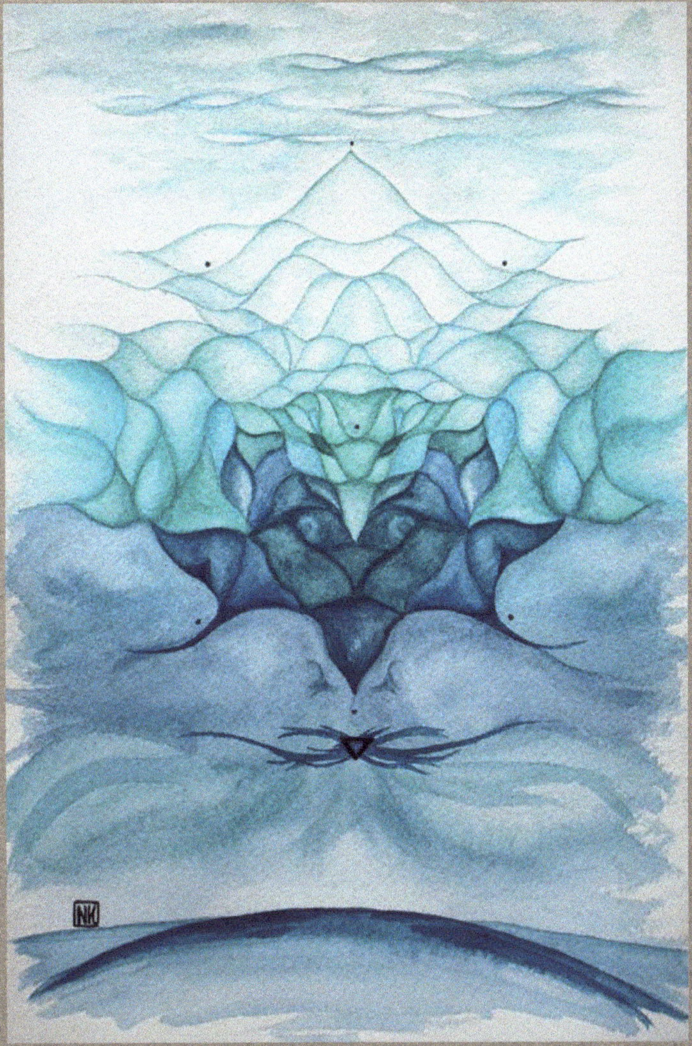

“Sri Aqua,” Watercolor © 2021 Nicole Rachelle Keane, Gratitude Healing Arts, LLC

"Continuous, calm, powerful use of the will shakes the forces of creation and brings a response from the infinite."

– Paramahansa Yogananda

THE CHARACTER FOR *PO*

魄

"Like the Chinese character *hun*, *po* contains the radical *gui* [on the right]...this character means 'earthbound spirit,' and is sometimes translated as 'ghost.' The top part represents the head of a person, while the bottom is the vaporous body of a spirit...the *gui* [are] ephemeral mists that float lightly about the surfaces of things...they are mysterious yet real, delicate and sensitive yet very powerful, and especially worthy of great respect...the radical *bai* [on the left], meaning 'white'..is a pictograph of the rising sun, the color white is associated with brightness and is related to the color of the eastern sky at dawn."

-Lori Eve Dachar, *'Five Spirits'*

Attributes of the Water Element

Spirit Affiliation - *po*

Organ officials: Kidney *yin,* Bladder *yang*

The purpose of *Water* is to flow. It is the great integrator; it receives, it disperses, it provides a fluid matrix for energy to move within. Our human form is made of water, as such energy travels through this fluid matrix within the physical form, as both wave and particle. At our highest manifestations, we are the embodiment of light.

The *po,* the spirit affiliation, and soul of *Water,* is referred to as the "Animal Wit," "Animal Soul," or "Corporeal Soul." It is the very human nature. Unlike the *hun* that linger on after our bodies return to the Earth, the *po* dies with us, vaporizing just as water sublimates, with the assistance of the heat of *Fire.*

Perhaps, if the light of the *hun,* and the strength of the *Fire* element, is not sufficient to vaporize the watery *po,* the fluid nature of our spirit, then our Corporeal Soul will be bound to another lifetime… As in the case of Ancestral Karma, entering through the Bladder meridian, the Uterus, and through to the *Water* element of the child at the time of birth. Within the wheel of Karma, the goal is to enlighten as much as possible through this lifetime, in order to eviscerate the *po* upon death…

An empty, light Heart, filled with the feathery grace of the *Shen* is essential for this practice of transmutation throughout life; when the Animal Soul passes, the Heart is said to be weighed against a feather, as the ancient Egyptians believed, on the scales of Anubis…

The two Soul spirits, the *hun* and the *po,* have an intimate relationship with each other. The *hun* and the *po* are both *yang* in nature, but the *po* is *yin* when related to the *hun*. I take this to mean that the *Po,* Soul aspect of the Spirit that is domicile within the Lungs, is *yin* in nature, and the *po* soul, the spirit affiliation of the *Water* element, is *yang* in nature.

The *Hun* (associated with the Triple Warmer and locations of Brown Adipose Tissue (BAT) throughout the body) and the *Po,* are linked by polarity. Anatomically, this is seen through the apex of the Lung where BAT is located. This is the location of the Upper Burner, above the clavicle, in the Thoracic Inlet. Notably, the *Hun* often reside in the Lesser Omentum, as mentioned previously, but do travel within the entire Triple Warmer complex of tissues and dispersed deposits of BAT.

The *hun* and the *po* are linked energetically within the *Tan Cycle* and *Yu Angles,* through the axis of the *Fire* element and the *Water* element; as well as through anatomical location of BAT near the Kidneys and the Urinary pathway.

Integration Potentials of the Water Element

The natural polarity of the holographic *Po/po,* or *yin/yang,* relationship is evident through the powerful integration and balancing potential of the *Water* element, and the ability of the Lungs to take in moisture and life force energy, and release vapor and toxins through the breath, coming into a sense of neutrality.

The *Po's* residence in the Lungs enable life to keep living; with every breath we take, we have the potential for animation and integration, to flow freely on our chosen path in life. The potential for re-animation also exists, through the power of the Lungs to activate the Ventral Vagal regulatory response through associations with its holographic potentials, represented within the *Water* element and the Sympathetic stress response, assisting in a shift away from Dorsal Vagal dominance and immobilization.

"The *Po* are the animating agents of vital life processes that take place beyond our conscious awareness and control." *(Dachar, Five Spirits)*

The *yang po* of the *Water* element are related to the seven emotions in Asian medical theory. Fear. Fright. Anger. Joy. Worry. Sadness. Grief.

These emotions stir the waters of our Soul, and activate the *po.* Oppression and Rumination are also considered emotions, but ones that stagnate the waters of the mind, causing the Heart to gradually fill and grow heavy, displacing the *Shen* toward the *Earth,* and reducing the power of the warmth that assists with the integration potentials of the *Water* element.

The animating, corporeal presence of the *po* is what connects us to our senses. It keeps us connected to the sacred space of our physical body and emotional experience.

The *po* is associated with the Sympathetic Nervous System (SNS). It is related to the emotions of Fear and fright, as well as reaction to touch, through energetic connection with the Dorsal Root ganglion of the spinal column, and the Sacral Sympathetic chain ganglion; both of which follow the Bladder meridian.

The *po's* nexus with the Parasympathetic Nervous System (PNS) involves the Sacral Parasympathetic, or Pelvic Splanchnic nerves.

The sensory experience of internal environment through the *po,* is associated with the concept of interoception, and the Parasympathetic Visceral Vagal afferent receptors.

This energetic connection within the *Water* element rests on the path of the Kidney Divergent channel, that ascends to meet with the Bladder Meridian, at the Dorsal Vagal Nuclei complex in the Medulla of the Brainstem. This complex receives afferent information from the viscera, relaying that information to higher order neurons and nuclei within the Limbic System, Basal Nuclei, and Cortex.

The *Zhi* Spirit, or Free Will, of the Kidneys, connects with its holographic counterpart, the *zhi* spirit affiliation of the *Wood* element, or Divine Will, when the Kidney Divergent channel meets with the Gallbladder meridian in this area of the Brain Stem, contributing to the orchestration of proper Autonomic balance through the Vagal Nuclei.

If the *po* of the *Water* element is unable to be supported by the Ventral Vagal regulatory system, and the Wisdom of the *zhi* within the *Wood* element, the human experience is one of Sympathetic arousal and a spectrum of anxiety.

The SNS qualities of "fight or flight," that we are so familiar with from historical concepts of the "stress reaction," are like a stream of turbid rapids rushing to the sea, or a wave breaking on the shore.

There is no ease. There is no grace. There is only survival.

Some psychoemotional characteristics of this type of stress response affecting the *po* of the *Water* element include:

- traits of "reacting" instead of "responding;"
- anxiety, the quality of which is related to extreme necessity for movement, or a sense of pressure building like steam;
- "running away" from relationships or difficult conversations;
- feeling as though you cannot respond or engage, with yourself or others, as if you are unable to connect internally with your desires and ideas, and holding words back; or
- feeling overwhelmed in situations, as if you were "drowning" in the experience.

The Sympathetic stress response is not only "fight or flight," but also can be characteristic of emotional and physical "bracing, holding, protecting, and flexing" behaviors, that are rooted in a need for control of one's internal and external environment. This is the inability to feel *safe* and have faith, or a trust in the process; there is an inability to receive the presence of flow.

Some physical aspects of a Sympathetic stress response with the qualities of *po* include:

- joint pain, or other pain that comes and goes;
- difficulty breathing, including symptoms of asthma;
- skin eruptions and rashes, eczema, or psoriasis patches;
- lipomas;
- fibroids;
- edema;
- withholding bodily functions, such as decreased urination and constipation; and
- increased urination.

Increased urination is often observed as an indicator of stress response, but may go unnoticed, or not attributed to stress. This happens, indirectly, due to up-regulation and activation of Vasopressin receptors; Vasopressin is also known as Anti-Diuretic Hormone (ADH), and is one of the key neurotransmitters referenced in the *Polyvagal Theory.* It is responsible for decreased urination in some circumstances, but also leads to an increase, in the case of chronic stress.

Release of Vasopressin happens during acute stress response to increase our blood pressure, in preparation for fight or flight. It also stimulates release of Adrenal Corticotropin Hormone (ACTH) from the Anterior Pituitary, which signals the release of Aldosterone from the Adrenal glands. Aldosterone is what increases urination when experiencing chronic stress that does not result in mobilization behavior.

This process may be modulated by the *Wood* element, and is directly related to the balance between the Gallbladder meridian and the Governing Vessel meridian.

Points and organs on both of these channels affect the emotional processing of the Limbic system, which affects the regulatory functions of the Hypothalamus, where Vasopressin is synthesized and released within the Hypophyseal portal, to affect the Anterior Pituitary.

These physical symptoms are a result of the *po* being weak because the *zhi,* or Divine Will, attributed to the *Wood* element, cannot lift and support the seat of Free Will, that is domicile within the Kidneys of the *Water* element. In other words, the Parasympathetic Ventral Vagal regulatory functions of the ANS are not strong enough to lift and support the natural Sympathetic response to stress.

A weakened *po,* that is not backed by a healthy Ventral Vagal regulatory response, may be attributed to physical and energetic restriction, going back further in the *Tan Cycle,* to the *Fire* element, and the *Hun,* nested in the Lesser Omentum.

Restrictions within the Lesser Omentum prevent free flow of accurate Vagal afferent information from the viscera to the Brainstem, through the Nodose Ganglia located within the Hepatic Hilum, and upper Hepatoduodenal ligament of the Lesser Omentum. As noted earlier, restrictions here can also prevent release of proper amounts of digestive enzymes from the Biliary tree and the Pancreas.

Tension in the Lesser Omentum can also cause a back up in fluids within the abdomen, creating edema and pressure around the Kidneys. This may affect the Diaphragm, creating tension from the physical restriction in the area, as well as the change in pressure differential between the Thorax and the Abdomen.

As the body adapts to allostatic load, or the physiological effects of the presence of chronic stress within the internal or external environment, energetic and physical tensions begin to build; the body has a response through interoception, and a resulting emotion, often on the spectrum of Fear.

The more chronic the stressor, and the more developed the trauma patterning within the nervous system, the more potential for physical and energetic examples of how the *hun* may not be able to lift and support the spirit of the *zhi*, leading to a backsliding in the *Tan Cycle*, affecting the *po* of the *Water* element, rendering it unable to lift and support the functions of the *Metal* element, causing weakness in the *Po* of the Lungs and the *yi*...and the immobilization response begins to unfold.

This backsliding within the *Tan Cycle*, and breakdown of the lifting and supporting functions of the *Five Elements*, is analogous to the concept of "dissolution" presented in the *Polyvagal Theory*.

"Dissolution is a construct introduced by the philosopher Herbert Spencer (1820-1903) to describe evolution in reverse. It was adapted by John Hughlings Jackson (1835-1911) to describe how brain damage, and brain disease, function similarly to a process of "de-evolution" in which evolutionarily older circuits become <u>dis</u>inhibited (Jackson, 1884). Polyvagal Theory adapts dissolution to explain the phylogenetically ordered hierarchy in which the Autonomic Nervous System responds with progressively evolutionarily older circuits." (*Porges, Polyvagal Theory)*

Interestingly, when *Water* is unable to lift and support *Metal* in solution, usually from too much heat, *Metal* will precipitate out of the solution (de-solution)…A similar process also happens as a function of cooling within the Sky.

When *Water* vapor reaches the dew point, as *Air* rises and encounters cooler temperatures, it condenses forming clouds; when the *Air* cools further, *Water* precipitates out of *Air* forming rain.

In this way, the relationship between the *Water* element, and the *Metal/Air* element is a very intimate one, and can be a bit volatile depending on physical (lack of blood flow, inflammation, connective tissue restrictions, ect.) and energetic (emotional) forms of hot and cold shifts, within the internal and external environment. These concepts of hot and cold (temperature control), can apply physically and energetically, to aspects of the *Fire* element, the spirit affiliation of *hun,* and Spirit of *Shen.*

The concept of dissolution within the *Five Elements*, relative to the *Polyvagal Theory*, is the initiation of a backsliding motion within the *Tan Cycle,* due to stress or trauma negatively affecting the spirit affiliations, resulting in a break down of support within the hierarchical, negentropic, system of the *Tan Cycle.*

Within this process of dissolution, the Parasympathetic Ventral Vagal regulatory functions associated with a healthy and balanced *Wood* element, are not able to appropriately manage the internal or external environmental stressor. This can be due to trauma history, physical or energetic restrictions on the meridian pathways, and innate physiology.

If the innate physiology of the person under stress or trauma cannot support a healthy return to Parasympathetic Ventral Vagal regulation, or if the Sympathetic response is not able to "fight or flight," the Parasympathetic Dorsal Vagal nervous system may be recruited in a last ditch effort for self preservation and survival.

This is akin to the *Tan Cycle* backsliding all the way to the *Metal* element, and can result in the energy of the person under stress turning to Stone, in a "freeze or feign" spectrum response.

This can manifest psychologically and physically through a myriad of symptoms including:

- depression,
- dissociation,
- immobilization reactions,
- twitching,
- fainting,
- black outs,
- acute abdominal pain,
- chronic pain such as fibromyalgia,
- chronic fatigue,
- chronic inflammation,
- autoimmune illness,
- breakdowns in the digestive processes,
- problems with blood pressure variability and regulation,
- low heart rate,
- low body temperature, and
- in extreme cases, bradycardia.

Physiologically, the Parasympathetic Dorsal Vagal reaction to stress or trauma is very hard to "get out of" because our human mammalian nervous system has no efficient pathway out of becoming the Stone.

We need to cognitively recruit our Sympathetic stress response, through the Prefrontal Cortex of the Bladder meridian, to step in for the immobilization response that is generated, as a survival technique, by our Dorsal Vagus.

Once we are able to be well regulated by the emotional awareness and physical balance of the Ventral Vagus, we are able to manifest the true path of our Soul in this life, free from the immobilization response of the Dorsal Vagus, and guided by the Divine Will of *zhi* and light of *hun*. The Animal Soul, and the Free Will of the *Zhi*, are now able to align with purpose toward the integration and evolution of our Self, adding to the Collective Consciousness.

When the *Wood* element is strong and able to support the *Water* element, the Sympathetic Nervous System can act in positive ways throughout the body; increasing blood flow; promoting growth and restoration, healing and renewal; and providing the energy for integration of physical and emotional trauma.

As discussed within the other spirit affiliations, the early childhood experiences one has significantly impact physiological and neurological resilience. Creating stability within the *Tan Cycle* is a process, and once a structure is set, you can heal some parts of it in this lifetime, if given the appropriate support. However, some aspects of this innate framework of one's nervous system may be more constitutional than others, and the energy needed to grow, to integrate, and to transform in *this* lifetime, may be very great. This is especially the case when relating to the deep, solid structures within the subconscious and how a personality is ordered.

In these cases, the interplay between *Water* and *Metal/Air* can lead to the transformation of subconscious patterning.

This type of transformation requires orchestration. It requires the help of the Divine guidance and spirit light of the *hun*, within the *Fire element*, as well as a healthy *Shen* population nested in the Heart, directing their light toward the *Zhi* or Free Will (Ego) within the Kidney, and the Animal Soul, the *Po*, of the Lungs within the *Metal* element. This interaction between *Fire-Water-Metal/Air* can be seen in the diagram of the *Yu Angles*, within the last section of this manual.

Just like the processes in the outward environment that create precipitation of *Metal* from *Water*, and *Water* from the *Air*, too much heat, or too much internal *Fire*, can lead to *Water* being unable to support *Metal*. Similarly, too little internal *Fire*, and a cool atmosphere above *Earth*, can lead to the *Air being* unable to support *Water*, in reciprocity, resulting in rain.

However, the right amount of warmth and a gentle, consistent light, from the *hun* and the *Shen*, can be very, *very* healing. Steady increases in temperature can lead to greater kinetic energy that allows for the solvent molecules, the *po* of *Water*, to more easily break apart the solute molecules that have a strong intermolecular attraction; in this case, *Water* has a greater capacity to suspend and support the spirit affiliation *yi* of the *Metal* element, our Consciousness of Potentials...and the innate structure, within the subconscious, of how we process emotional experiences.

Steady warmth and light assists the *Water* element with integration, this increases solubility... and convection...both processes of integration.

The Resilience of *po*

Within the character for *po,* is the symbol for 'white,' the quality of the light of the Moon and the silvering of the shadows at night.

The symbol for *gui* is relative to the dark sides of our Ego, the potent mix of our Animal Soul, the *po,* and the Free Will, Egoic, aspects of the Spirit *Zhi.* The resilience, and brilliance, of the *Water* element can be found where the light of the Moon illuminates the shadows of our Soul.

Human nature has a shadow side that is created by experience and time. When we give enough pause in the daily flow of our lives to reflect on the image of our Shadow in the waters before us, we are able to participate in a process of awareness that will lead to our ultimate renewal.

When we are triggered by trauma, or drama, or stress in our lives, if we are able to stop and reflect on our reactions, with the Wisdom and equanimity of an aligned *zhi*, from a vantage point within a stable and balanced *Wood* element, the regulatory functions of our Ventral Vagus are able to calm and reason with our Animal Soul. This lifts and supports our ability to process and respond appropriately, so we do not slip into a reactionary state of Sympathetic stress or Dorsal Vagal immobilization.

In this way, we are able to break the cycle of trauma, and reunite the Divine Will, the *zhi,* of the *Wood* element, with the Free Will, Spirit *Zhi*, domiciled within the Kidneys. It is here where we may lean on the integrative powers of the *Water* element, and renew ourselves with our Divine nature, guided by the *hun* and the light of the *Shen.*

The shadow Self must be integrated and renewed, within the element of *Water*, for this alignment to happen in a gentle, non re-traumatizing way... this is done most gently with the lifting and supporting nature of the *Wood* element...just as the silvery light of a full Moon is filtered through the leaves of a tree.

On a physiological level, too much heat or light from the *Fire* element, too much emotion, leads to lack of reason in processing, as the energy of *Fire* bypasses the lifting and supporting properties of *Wood (Ventral Vagus)*, and creates an assault on the *Water* element, taking the Frontal lobe of the Brain along the Bladder meridian, our cognitive processing potential, offline.

This often leads to more trauma, or drama, and activation of the Sympathetic Nervous System (SNS). This is how neural impulses originating in the emotional enters of the Brain: the Limbic System, activating the HPA axis of the Hypothalamus, Pituitary, and Adrenal glands. These structures then interact with the Basal nuclei in the Brain, along the Bladder Meridian, to initiate movement through the Peripheral Nervous System... actualizing fight or flight response.

This kinetic energy, that has been created within the SNS, needs to flow out of the body through being transferred into movement. If the energy is not physiologically transferred, backsliding within the *Tan Cycle* occurs, and a shift into Parasympathetic Dorsal Vagal pathology happens, resulting in physical and emotional symptoms on the spectrum of immobilization. Within the *Water* element, as well as the *Metal/Air* element, the allostatic load of stress can also signal acute Sacral Parasympathetic responses, and potentially symptoms of Vasovagal reflex, spontaneous urination or defecation, and syncope.

Returning to Flow

The primal nature of the *po* is an embodiment of resilience. Movement is essential for the discharge of emotional energy from the body.

In order to return to a state of flow and integration; to be able to access the lifting and supporting rhythm of the Ventral Vagus through the *Wood* element, a focus must be shifted to the Root, so the *Water* may rise to the Branch.

The Sacral chakra, or the Sacral plexus, is associated with the *Water* element. This area is neurologically tied to the Sympathetic Nervous System (SNS), Adrenals, Genitourinary system, and last part of the Large Intestine (from the Sigmoid Colon down), as well as the Parasympathetic Sacral Splanchnic nerves; this illustrates another nexus between the *Water* and *Metal/Air* elements.

In order to initiate a return to flow through the *Wood* element, the Sacral chakra must recruit the Root chakra, just as the roots of a tree engage *Water*, and initiate a pumping action to slowly raise *Water* from its resting place within the substrate of *Metal* and *Earth*.

Linking the Breath with contractions of the Pelvic floor, assists in a rise of the *Water* element. Breathing low into the Lungs, with a relaxed Diaphragm; then extending the out breath, while simultaneously contracting the Diaphragm and Pelvic floor, is a very powerful *Way* to initiate a restoration. Repeating this sequence in a flowing pattern, like waves, will stimulate a healthy Sympathetic response, and assist in lifting the Spirit from an immobilization reflex or reaction.

In my experience, I have found that it is good to follow this exercise with movement of some sort: walking, tai chi, dancing, ect...however One is able to comfortably move. It is important to integrate movement that is not stressful to the physical body.

Any playful movement that can be easily accessed within One's physical ability, followed by a resting phase of calm, will help shift the body, as the Parasympathetic Ventral Vagal regulatory system takes over for the SNS. Balance of the emotions and the ANS can be achieved much more easily from this place, than when in a state of immobilization or emotional shut down.

The Root chakra and the Sacral chakra are very much linked neurologically. Recruiting the muscles of the Pelvic floor activates the *Wood* element by engaging the Liver Divergent channel and Gallbladder meridian, as well as the Vagus nerve.

The Vagus sends Parasympathetic fibers all the way down to the genital area. In this way, recruiting the Pelvic floor muscles helps increase Vagal tone, through energetically engaging the *Wood* element, just as the Xylem within trees contract to lift *Water* from the Roots, into circulation within the matrix of *Wood*.

Both energetic and physical, movement is essential for the resilience of the human body and Soul. The human body and Soul need movement in order to integrate our experience, and return from a state of being frozen in Stone, such as when there is backsliding through the *Tan Cycle,* and entropic processes of overwhelm or dissolution.

Even the simple act of shaking or wiggling can be enough to stir the Roots of the Autonomic Nervous System to respond in a healthy way.

Finding a neurologic path to resilience in the landscape of debilitating stress or intense trauma, can sometimes be hard, as we try our best to see through the fog; in these times, we must instead feel through the fog, by returning to our Body through gentle, supportive motion.

Physical vibration is energetic vibration, like the singing of a crystal bowl; the harmonics create waves within our fluid fascial matrix on a quantum level.

And like *Water*, in waves, we begin to Rise.

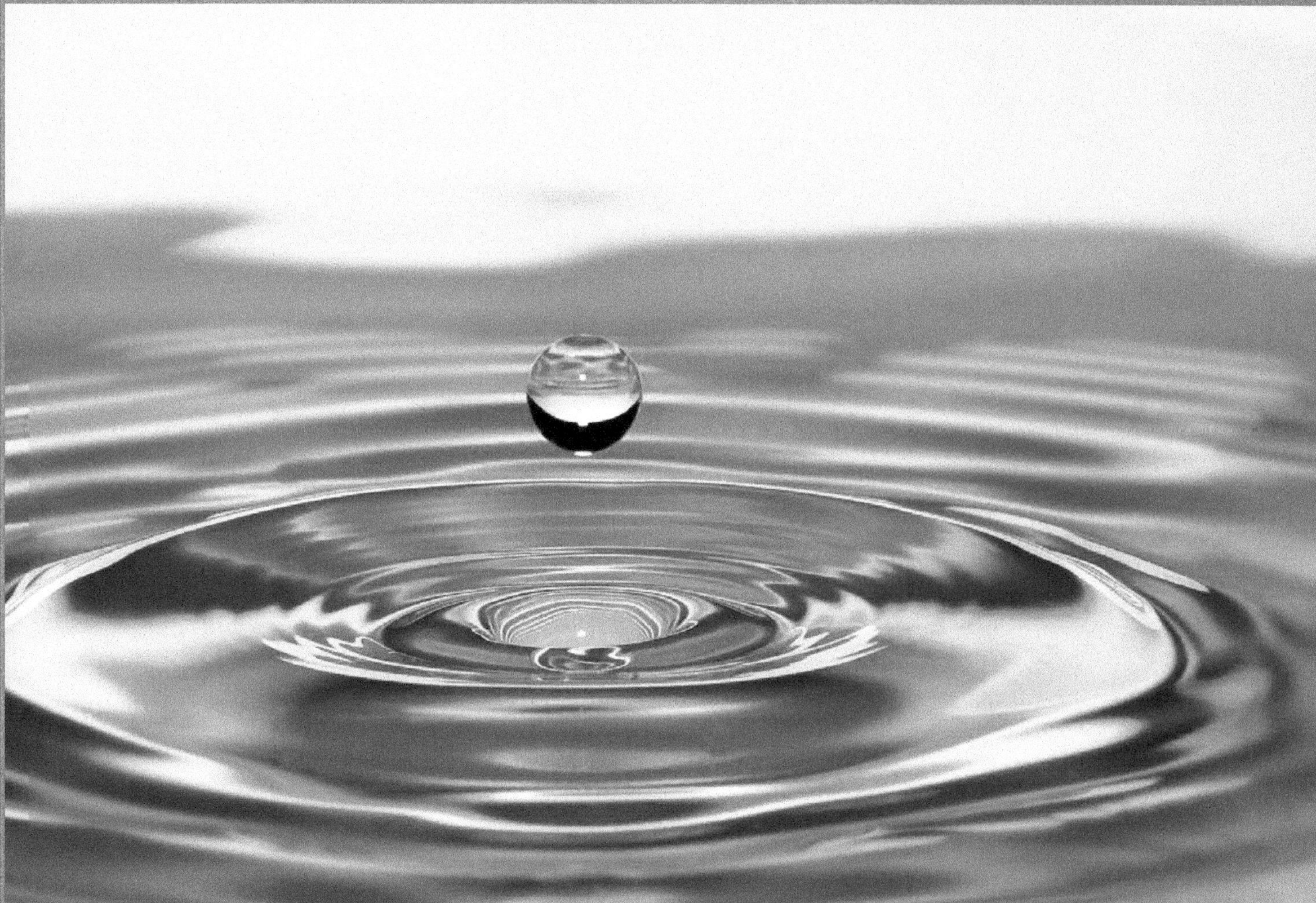

"And so we lift our gazes not to what stands between us, but what stands before us.

We close the divide because we know to put our future first, we must first put our differences aside."

- Amanda Gorman, "The Hill We Climb"

Practical Application of the *Tan Cycle*

The material and ideas that have been presented in this manual are meant as a reformation proposal for traditional *Five Element* theory, and to be used as a guide within the shifting energies that are unfolding and evolving among the Collective.

We are within the beginning stages of a dramatic paradigm shift. Just as the *Polyvagal Theory* has been revolutionary to the understanding of how trauma affects the human Autonomic Nervous System, I hope the thoughts presented here evoke a wider frame of view, toward the potentials of a world of modern physical and emotional healing, rooted in a knowing that is accessible to us all; a knowing that is only growing in awareness as we renew our connection with our environment.

As one Observes and learns any skill, the initial formal education is just a license to learn more. We learn the most from the experiences offered as a new knowing expands our lives through practice.

The practice of anything, especially medicine and healing, is just that; it is a practice; it is a process; it is an evolution; it is a revolution of Wisdom. We are within an era of evolutionary leaps in every direction. We are within an array of new beginnings. This manual is part of that unfolding; it is just another beginning in the renewal process of what has always been known within.

There no longer needs to be such division between modern medicine of the "West," and ancient knowing of the "East."

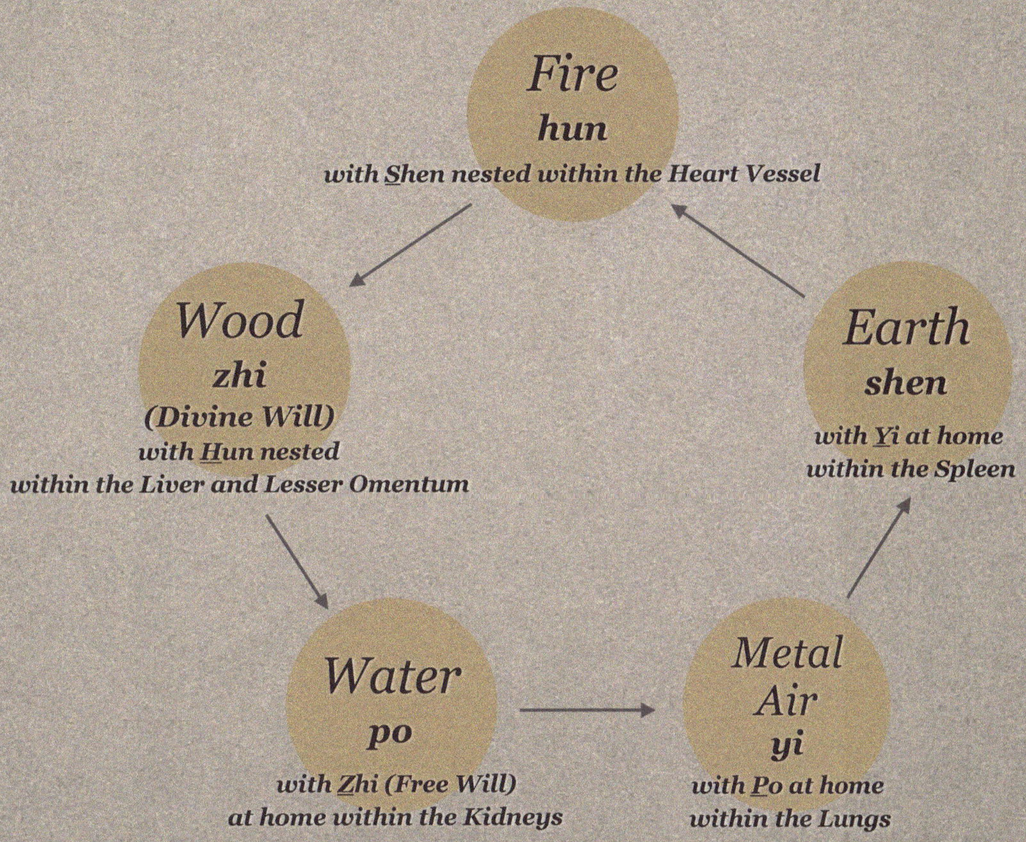

THE *TAN CYCLE*
THE *TRANSFORMATIONAL CYCLE* OF THE *RENEWED SPIRIT AFFILIATIONS*

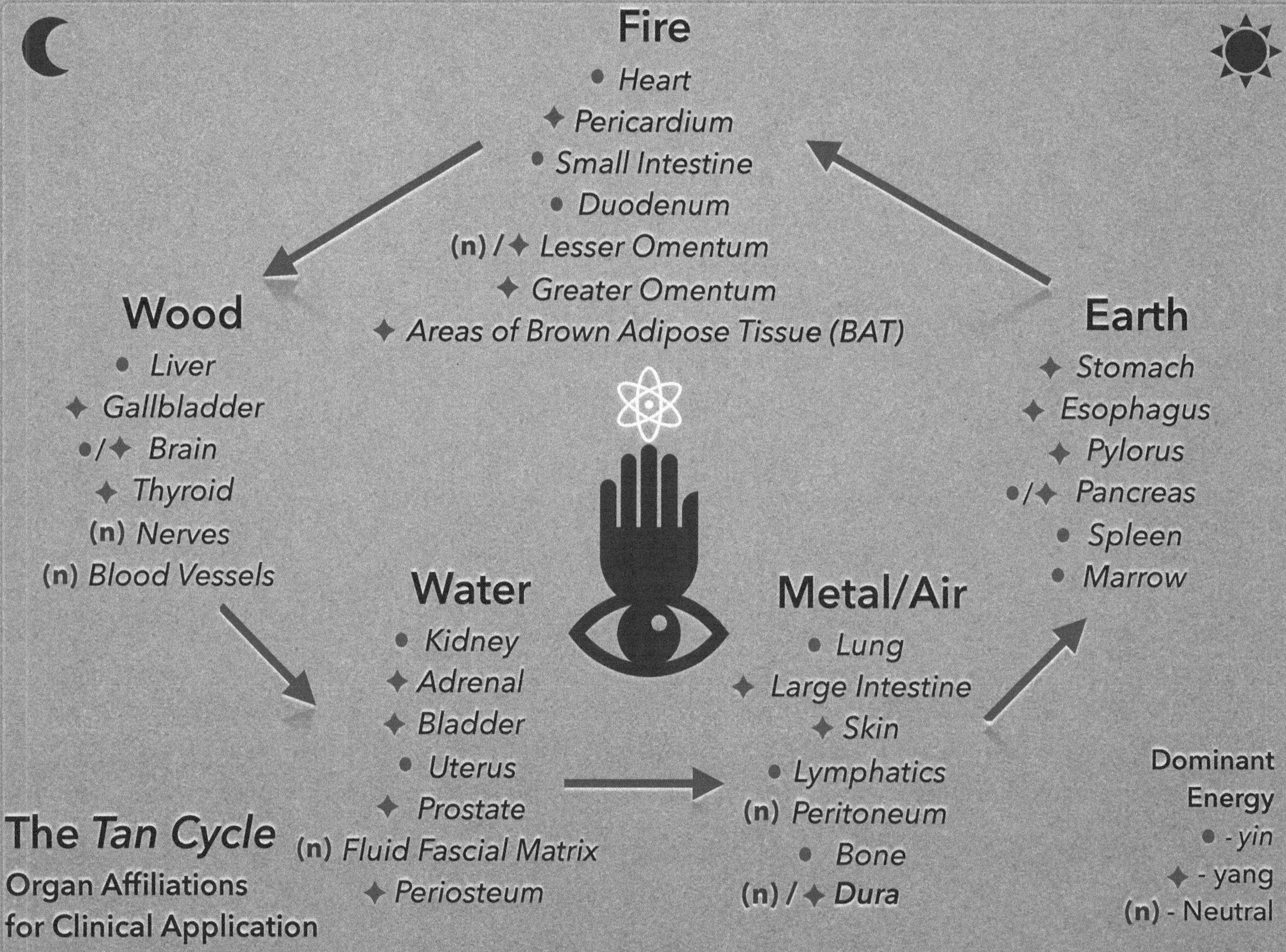
Fire
• Heart
✦ Pericardium
• Small Intestine
• Duodenum
(n) / ✦ Lesser Omentum
✦ Greater Omentum
✦ Areas of Brown Adipose Tissue (BAT)
Wood
• Liver
✦ Gallbladder
•/✦ Brain
✦ Thyroid
(n) Nerves
(n) Blood Vessels
Earth
✦ Stomach
✦ Esophagus
✦ Pylorus
•/✦ Pancreas
• Spleen
• Marrow
Water
• Kidney
✦ Adrenal
✦ Bladder
• Uterus
✦ Prostate
(n) Fluid Fascial Matrix
✦ Periosteum
Metal/Air
• Lung
✦ Large Intestine
✦ Skin
• Lymphatics
(n) Peritoneum
• Bone
(n) / ✦ Dura
Dominant Energy
• - yin
✦ - yang
(n) - Neutral
The Tan Cycle
Organ Affiliations for Clinical Application

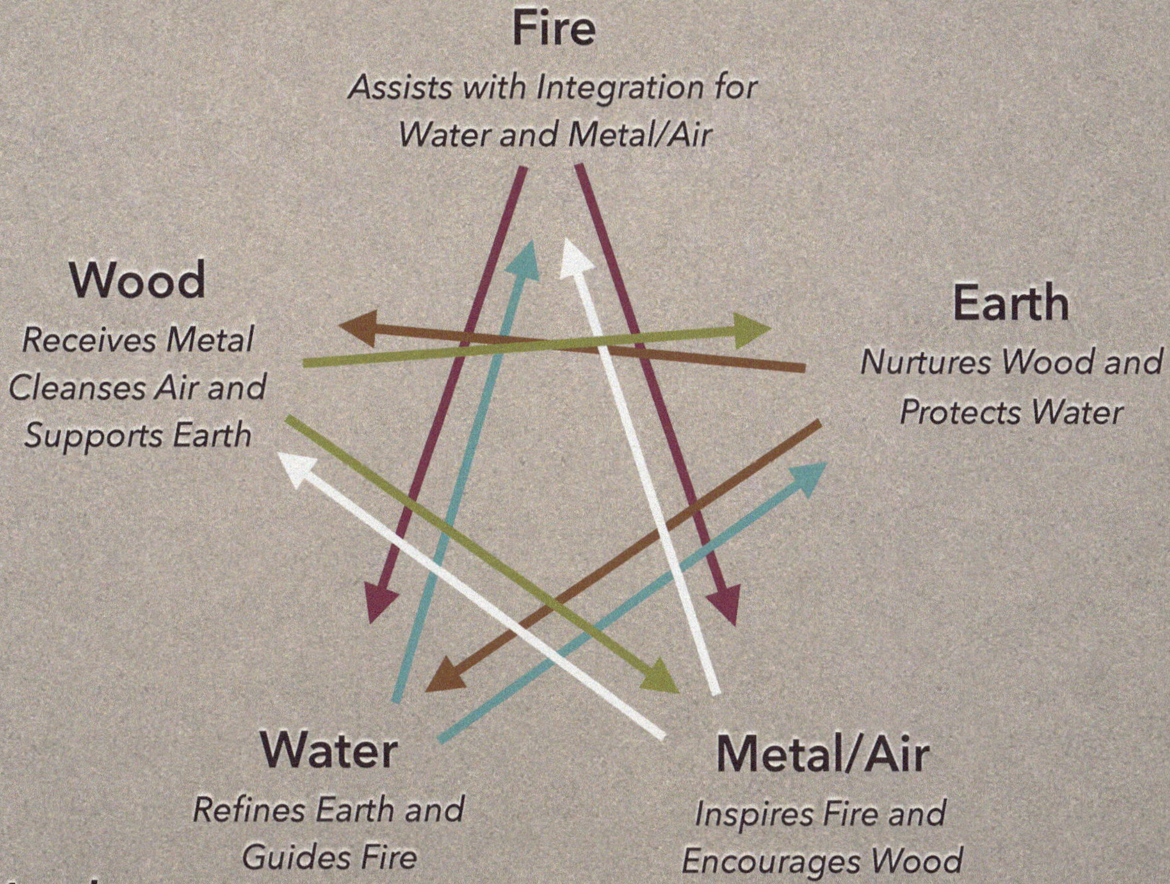

The *Yu Angles*

Elemental Associations
for Clinical Application

The *Tan Cycle,* and the concept of the renewed spirit affiliations, are meant to be integrated into an existing practice, and expanded upon in ways the Observer sees appropriate. This is a guide toward a path, and an introduction to a *Way* of learning through listening to the Body.

When encountering symptoms that fit into characteristics of one of the *Five Elements,* I ask that the Observer pause and take a moment to consider the concepts presented in this manual. How may the symptoms be a manifestation of the nervous system having had an experience of trauma or stress? Could these symptoms be a potential disturbance of Autonomic resilience?

I ask you, as an Observer, to consider how you may look past the symptom; look past the established patterns and environment that created the imbalance; and look toward what may be required to rebuild resilience from a place of support.

As a general rule, although of course there may be some exceptions, if there is physical or energetic disfunction within the *yin* organ, meridian line, or Divergent channel, of a particular element where the Spirit is domicile; then the Observer would look toward the *yang* organ of the preceding element within the *Tan Cycle* for potentials of energetic or physical restriction that may be disrupting, or distorting the ability of that *yang* energy to lift and support the *yin* energy.

For example, if there is a symptom associated with the *yin* organ and energetic pathways of the *Water* element, one would look toward the organ and channels of the *yang* energy of the *Wood* element, to lift and support the *Water* element. In this way, the holographic spirit affiliation, the *zhi* of the *Wood* element, is always in relationship to its Spirit that is domicile in the physical *yin* organ of the *Water* element; wave and particle, energetic and physical… together, on the path of healing.

This "rule" applies, but for the placement of the *Hun,* which has somewhat of a dispersed residence in the tissues of the Triple Warmer. When in balance, the *Hun* is found near the tissues of the Lesser Omentum and the Liver. The duel organ affiliations within the *Fire* element may also challenge the application of this theory. In these areas, I encourage the Observer to get creative, and use the principles offered in this manual to perfect their healing art.

Now, if there is physical or energetic restriction within the *yang* organ, meridian line, or Divergent channel, of a particular element, the Observer would look first to its elemental paired *yin* organ for disfunction, or distortion, within the physical structure, or energy channels; as it is likely the *yin* energy may be unable to support the *yang* from a place of grace.

In this way, the polarity of Feminine and Masculine, or *yin* and *yang,* of a particular element, are always in relationship to each other. Likewise, a chain of energetic distortion can be followed and mended along the *Way*, as previously referenced through the *Tan Cycle.*

Treatment through this protocol with in the *Tan Cycle* is a "direct" Way of treatment, which may or may not be appropriate for those with a traumatic past, pattern of chronic stress, or anyone in a process of rebuilding resilience.

For additional healing potentials that are more "indirect," and to augment the counter-clockwise flow of *qì* within the *Tan Cycle,* consideration of the *Yu Angles* is very important. Treatment from this perspective is far less likely to retraumatize a system than most direct interventions.

As seen in the figure referencing the *Yu Angles,* the Observer would look toward the two elements at *Yu Angles* from the element of focus, from the element that is most descriptive of the symptom at hand. Assessing and treating these elements for energetic and physical restrictions within the specific organs, tissues, meridian lines, and Divergent channels, will offer the most gentle support and assistance toward restoring the counter-clockwise flow of *qì* within the system.

Using *Yu Angles* is particularly effective in situations where there has been a complex, or chronic, trauma history, because treating the elements at *Yu Angles* from a symptom offers a "back door" to working with the nervous system, and can affect the energetic and emotional balance from a place of ease, rather than working directly with the preceding element within the *Tan Cycle,* which may be too much, too soon, in some cases.

Moreover, as in the case where the *Fire* element interacts with the integration aspects of the *Water* and *Metal/Air* elements, if there is a disturbance that can be seen as a cluster of symptoms characteristic of two adjacent elements, the Observer would look toward the element that assists them both, within the *Yu Angles,* for an efficient option to initiate healing.

It is not my intention to confuse those already practicing *Five Element* theory with this philosophy and these treatment theories, only to open the Observer to a possibility that intuitively resonates on a level that was previously out of reach of the Collective. As our knowledge about the Body and Mind evolves, so too will our innate awareness.

The information presented in this manual is meant for application by an Observer, rooted in a place that is open; with good boundaries; and the clarity of *pu*, the uncarved block; an Observer that is able to listen to the Body and Spirit that is before them, without projection or clouded perception.

These theories can be applied to manual therapies, or purely energetic work such as needle based acupuncture; however, I find in my practice: there is no substitute for direct contact with the tissues of the body...as long as the practitioner is in a well regulated, balanced emotional state, within a healing atmosphere that is *rooted in a sense of safety.*

"It is through our own authenticity, our own willingness to embody our natural vibration, that we can resonate with all things. When we can be in this space, we are simultaneously individual and collective. In this Mind-field, we can begin to communicate through resonance, to harmonize. This is the energy of the solution consciousness."

– Peter Shea, 'Alchemy of the Extraordinary'

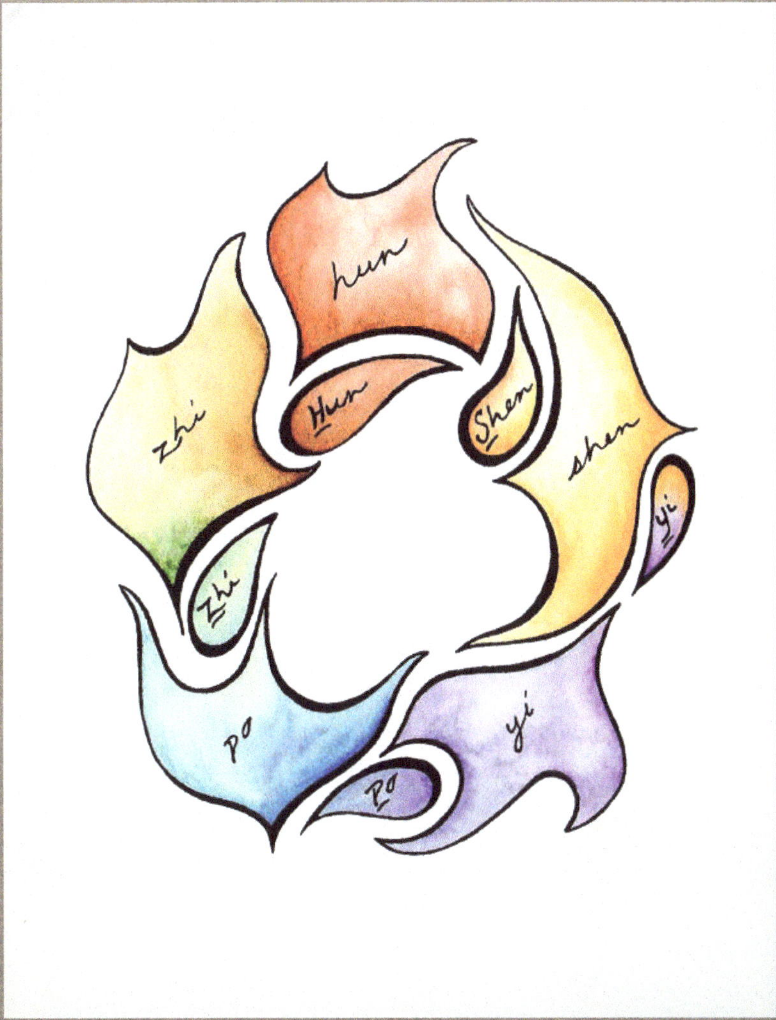

"The Holographic Nature of the Spirit Affiliations"
Ink and Watercolor © 2021 Nicole Rachelle Keane, Gratitude Healing Arts, LLC

Elemental Manual Meridian Theory and Techniques (EMMT)

If you would like to learn more about the anatomy, physiology, and manual therapy techniques, relative to the *Polyvagal Theory* and application of the *Tan Cycle*, I have created a curriculum called Elemental Manual Meridian Theory and Techniques (EMMT). These EMMTs are intended to be clinical applications of the *Polyvagal Theory*, within the structure of the *Five Element* theory that is presented in this manual.

The material that I present through the EMMT courses, will offer an awareness of how to expand upon current healing practices in new and dynamic ways. This curriculum will clarify historical concepts of *Five Element* Asian medical theory, and create a space that will open the Mind to alternate perspectives.

I have tried to make the material presented in the EMMT courses easily accessible by offering:

- classes in pre-recorded, learn at your own pace modules;
- detailed description of the anatomy, and related physiology, of primary organs, curious organs, primary meridian channels, and channel divergencies;
- licensed images from the Netter Atlas of Human Anatomy, Seventh Edition;
- access to a PDF of the study manual, and all audio/visual presentation modules; as well as
- opportunities for additional in person, hands on, mentorship sessions.

The curriculum presented in the EMMT courses is based on manual contact with the tissues of the body, in alignment with the concepts of Neuroception and Interoception. It is a trauma informed practice, based on a treatment theory that is inherently supportive and safe, leading to a gentle, powerful, sovereign, and non-retraumatizing experience.

The EMMT curriculum is taught in a series of 5 classes (*Wood, Fire, Earth, Metal/Air, and Water*). The *Polyvagal Theory* will be the foundation for this curriculum, and will be used to relate how manual therapy, within the *Five Elements*, directly affects the Autonomic Nervous System (ANS) and Vagus nerve complex. Techniques in these classes will blend together:

- Toyohari Style Meridian Therapy,
- Visceral Mobilization,
- Neural Mobilization,
- Circulatory Release Techniques,
- Myofascial Release,
- Structural Integration Theory, and
- Lymphatic Drainage, with an awareness of:
- Neuroendocrine Balancing, and
- Identification of Emotional Holding Patterns.

The curriculum begins with the *Wood* element class, as this is a critical class in the EMMT series, due to its energetic and anatomical relationship to the Vagus nerve complex. Each class in this series will build on the next, as the whole is greater than the sum of its parts!

I ask that the Observer always hold an awareness of what resonates within themselves along the path of learning and exploring this material. If manual therapy is not included as part of your scope of practice, these courses will still be interesting to all, and provide ideas for integrating this type of therapy into current and future plans of care, through referrals to other providers.

The combination of the *Polyvagal Theory,* with the evolved aspects of *Five Element* theory, as applied to modern knowledge of anatomy, physiology, and psychology, offers a truly alchemical, as well as efficient, healing potential.

The objective of the Observer should be to meet the Body, and Spirit, wherever it is, and show it the *Way* to resilience through following a path of *safety* and support.

If you are interested in exploring more, please visit: www.gratitudehealingarts.com.

RESOURCES AND RECOMMENDED READING

Chödrön, Pema. When Things Fall Apart: Heart Advice for Difficult Times. Boston: Shambhala; 2000.

Chödrön, Pema. The Wisdom of No Escape: And the Path of Loving-Kindness. Boston; London; 2001.

Lighthorse, Pixie. Goldmining The Shadows. Lighthorse Publishing. 2019

Dechar, Lorie Eve. Five Spirits: Alchemical Acupuncture for Psychological and Spiritual Healing. Lantern Books; 2006.

Laozi, ., & Mitchell, S. (1988). Tao Te Ching: A new English Version. New York, N.Y: Harper & Row.

Wilhelm, R., Jung, C. G., & Baynes, C. F. The Secret of the Golden Flower, A Chinese Book of Life, Translated and Explained by Ricard Wilhelm, with a European commentary by C.G. Jung; with eleven plates and four text illustrations. London: K. Paul, Trench, Trubner & Co.. 1935

Shea, Peter. Alchemy of the Extraordinary: A Journey into the Heart of the Meridian Matrix. Soul Pivot Press; 2015.

Dolowich, Gary. Archetypal Acupuncture: Healing with the Five Elements. Jade Mountain Publishing; 2003.

Farrell, Yvonne R. Psycho-Emotional Pain and the Eight Extraordinary Vessels. Singing Dragon; 2016.

Duncan, Alaine D; Kain, Kathy L. The Tao of Trauma: A Practitioner's Guide for Integrating Five Element Theory and Trauma Treatment. North Atlantic Books; 2019.

Kaptchuk, T. J. The Web That Has No Weaver. Contemporary Books; 2000.

Jarrett, Lonny. Nourishing Destiny: The Inner Tradition of Chinese Medicine. Spirit Path Press; 2015.

Porges SW. The Polyvagal Perspective. Biol Psychol. 2007;74(2):116-143. doi:10.1016/j.biopsycho.2006.06.009

Porges SW. The Pocket Guide to the Polyvagal Theory: The Transformative Power of Feeling Safe. W.W. Norton; 2017.

Porges SW. The Polyvagal Theory Neurophysiological Foundations of Emotions, Attachment, Communication, and Self-Regulation. W.W. Norton; 2011.

Marlien, Eric. A New Approach to the Vagus Nerve and Autonomic Nervous System. Barral Productions; 2021.

Netter, Frank H. Altas of Human Anatomy. 5th Ed. Saunders, Elsevier Inc; 2011.

Kahn-John Diné M, K'oithan M. Living In Health, Harmony, and Beauty: The Diné (Navajo) Hózhó Wellness Philosophy. Glob Adv Health Med. 2015;4(3):24-30. doi:10.7453/gahmj.2015.044